Introduction to
Adult
Swallowing
Disorders

Michael A. Crary, Ph.D.
Florida Dysphagia Institute
University of Florida Health Science Center
Gainesville, Florida

Michael E. Groher, Ph.D.
Florida Dysphagia Institute
University of Florida Health Science Center
Gainesville, Florida

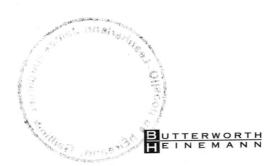

BUTTERWORTH
HEINEMANN

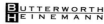

BUTTERWORTH
HEINEMANN

An Imprint of Elsevier Science

11830 Westline Industrial Drive
St. Louis, Missouri 63146

Introduction to Adult Swallowing Disorders   ISBN 0-7506-9995-7
Copyright © 2003, Elsevier Science (USA). All rights reserved.

Notice

Publishing Director: Linda Duncan
Acquisitions Editor: Kellie White
Developmental Editor: Jennifer Watrous
Project Manager: Joy Moore
Designer: Amy Buxton

Printed in the United States of America
Last digit is the print number: 9 8 7 6 5 4 3

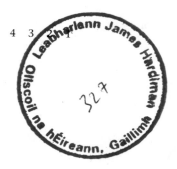

P R E F A C E

During the past 15 years, rehabilitation specialists, including speech pathologists, occupational therapists, physical therapists, and dietitians have combined their efforts in the care of persons with swallowing disability. In medical settings, 70% to 80% of patients composing a speech pathologist's caseload are persons with swallowing disorders. Speech pathologists have taken the lead in providing the research base that has led to the successful clinical management of dysphagic patients. Many speech pathologists have become leaders of interdisciplinary teams that interact to provide the most effective care to those with swallowing dysfunction. In most cases, the training necessary to manage the dysphagic patient is acquired by exposure at a clinical site treating patients with swallowing dysfunction. Few training institutions offer entire courses in the care of the swallowing-impaired patient, and even fewer have clinical sites where students can demonstrate their knowledge. This book is written with the intent of involving the novice rehabilitation specialist, particularly the speech pathologist, at a basic, introductory level of preparation. In our opinion, the lack of an introductory text has delayed and fragmented the basic preparation needed in a subspeciality of speech pathology that is the fastest growing segment of our total patient population.

The book provides chapters in both diagnostic and treatment domains, establishing the bridges between the two that are necessary for successful patient management. Diagnostic applications include chapters on epidemiology, the normal swallow, characteristics of common disorders, and physical and instrumental examination techniques. The treatment chapters focus on treatment selection, implementation, and measurement. Key points of diagnosis and treatment will be illustrated by the use of an accompanying videotape that include videofluoroscopic and endoscopic examples of normal and abnormal swallowing sequences and examples of the effects of treatment maneuvers on swallowing physiology (see accompanying videotape, Crary and Groher, *Video Introduction to Adult Swallowing Disorders*, Butterworth-Heinemann).

For teaching ease, each chapter begins with questions that should help focus the reader on a conceptual overview of the central issues relevant to the topic of discussion. Unfamiliar terminology is highlighted within the chapter and defined at the chapter's end. Also included at the end of each chapter are summary statements (Take Home Notes) that can be used to focus class discussion or as specific reminders of the most important content. Case examples also are provided to help the student integrate the basic concepts from each chapter.

It is our hope that the organization and introductory level of the chapters and the accompanying videotape will facilitate the teaching of students new to the concepts involved in managing dysphagic persons. Until now, no text has been designed specifically with this group of students in mind. In many respects, the practice has led the theory, spawning texts at a more advanced level, forgetting that the demand for entry level practitioners is continuing to grow.

The accompanying videotape includes normal and abnormal examples of the two most commonly used laboratory tests of swallowing function, endoscopy and videofluoroscopy. We chose to illustrate abnormalities not by diagnosis, but by the types of physiologic impairment one might encounter. It is our opinion that for the novice, linking specific diagnoses to videofluorographic or endoscopic results may be misleading and counterproductive to an understanding of their interpretation. In chapters there are liberal references to the videotape as a means to enhance the text.

In keeping with the concept of an introductory text, we have kept the terminology simple but relevant. The topics in chapters are comprehensive but not exhaustive. The overall content is straightforward for ease of learning, yet it is provocative and challenging for retention of learning. Specific book and journal article references in chapters have been kept at a minimum for ease of reading. Each chapter is followed by a list of suggested readings that support each chapter's content.

In general, we have tried to offer a text that entices the novice in a way that makes him or her feel not overwhelmed but comfortable with a new and exciting arena of health care. It is our hope that the outcome of this work will allow the student to enter an unfamiliar area confidently, with a solid base of knowledge that stems from research and experiential applications that help guide clinical decisions. Our goal has been to communicate a process of how clinical decisions are made in the care of dysphagic persons.

CONTENTS

C H A P T E R   1

Swallowing Disorders: An Overview

FOCUS QUESTIONS

1 What is dysphagia?
2 How does the knowledge of the incidence or prevalence of a disorder aid in the detection of dysphagia?
3 What major diagnoses precipitate dysphagia?
4 What are the differences in the types of patients seen at different levels of patient care? How does this affect the swallowing disorders specialist?
5 Who are potential members of the swallowing team? What are their roles?

DEFINITION

Dysphagia is the medical term used to describe a swallowing disorder. It is correctly pronounced with a long or short *a*. The final syllable, *ja*, requires a hard pronunciation rather than the soft *dja* to avoid confusion with the language disorder, *dysphasia*.

Medical students learn that dysphagia is a swallowing problem primarily associated with disease of the esophagus. However, used properly, the term *dysphagia* may refer to a swallowing disorder involving any one of the three stages of swallowing: oral, pharyngeal, or esophageal. It is not a primary medical diagnosis, but is a symptom of a disease, and therefore is described most often by its clinical characteristics.

Dysphagia is a delay in, or misdirection of, a fluid or solid food bolus as it moves from the mouth to the stomach. Delay or misdirection of the food bolus may interfere with functional oral intake. A swallowing disorder must be distinguished from a feeding disorder. A feeding disorder is an impairment in the process of food transport outside of the alimentary system. A feeding disorder usually is the result of weakness or incoordination in the arm used to move the food from the plate to the mouth. In some countries, a feeding disorder, particularly in the context of infants and children, is the same as a swallowing disorder. Persons with feeding disorders (motor transfer problems) also may be dysphagic (e.g., persons with cerebral palsy whose neurologic disability affects both feeding and swallowing). It is not known whether a feeding disorder that might necessitate assistance with food transport also affects the subsequent act of swallowing.

INCIDENCE/PREVALENCE

The *incidence* of a disorder is the reported frequency of new occurrences of that disorder over a long period (usually at least 1 year) in relation to the population in which it occurs. The *prevalence* of a disorder is the number of cases in a population during a shorter, prescribed period, usually in a specific setting. Most of the reported demographic data relating to swallowing disorders are prevalence data. Knowledge of the prevalence of a disorder is important, because it can help guide clinicians in the detection of that disorder, and therefore helps the clinician plan how resources might be devoted to that disorder. For example, if an examiner knows that a certain abnormality is found in less than 1% of a population, the examiner may not spend time looking for that abnormality, because its expected frequency of occurrence is low. However, if a particular abnormality is found in more than 50% of the persons with a particular disorder, the examiner is alerted to expect the occurrence of deficits associated with that disorder. Therefore if the data suggests that 30% of the patients suffering from acute stroke are dysphagic, an examiner expects that swallowing will be impaired in 3 of 10 acute stroke patients.

Some authors have estimated that the incidence of dysphagia in adults in the United States is 6%. Kuhlemeier reported that the incidence of reported dysphagia in the state of Maryland is 10 in 1000. The incidence of esophageal dysfunction was found to be 22.3% in 55-year-old Swedes. If these data are reliable, dysphagia is a common symptom. Dysphagia is seen most often in hospital and nursing home care settings. Dysphagia is most common in persons with neurologic disease (e.g., stroke, head injury, Parkinson's disease) and in those who have been treated for head and neck cancer.

Stroke

Prevalence reports of dysphagia following stroke depend on when in the course of recovery the detection of a swallowing impairment was made. For instance, in patients with acute stroke (less than 5 days after onset), the prevalence of dysphagia may be as high as 50%, whereas 2 weeks after stroke the prevalence may be only 10% to 28%. Recognizing these discrepancies, Smithard et al. followed 121 (untreated) acute stroke patients for 6 months using a clinical dysphagia examination and **videofluoroscopy** to detect swallowing deficits. Immediately following stroke, 51% were thought to be at risk for **aspiration**. After 7 days, only 27% were still considered at risk. At 6 months, 8% had persistent difficulty, whereas 3% who previously were not dysphagic were now considered at risk. These results suggest that early detection is important in preventing dysphagic complications and that a significant number of patients improve without intervention specific to their dysphagia. Daniels et al. found that 21 of 55 patients (38%) with acute stroke aspirated. Of these, two thirds did so silently (i.e., events of aspiration could be detected only by videofluoroscopy, not by the bedside examination). In long-term follow up, 94% of these patients returned to oral intake. Interestingly, the presence or absence of **silent aspiration** did not discriminate between patients who successfully returned to oral feeding.

Because of the bilateral innervation of the volitional muscles of deglutition, traditional theories of neuropathology suggest that dysphagia following neurologic insult to the motor pathways results only from bilateral disease. For instance, Horner et al. found that in 70 patients referred for dysphagia and suspected aspiration, 49% had bilateral brain insults. However, unilateral hemispheric and subcortical strokes also may result in significant dysphagic complications. Hamdy et al. studied a large series of unilateral stroke patients for several months. At initial presentation, 70% were dysphagic. At 3 months, 40% remained dysphagic as confirmed by videofluorographic studies. These results refute the concept that only bilateral stroke can produce dysphagia and that dysphagia from unilateral stroke is transitory. (See Chapter 4 for a complete discussion of neurogenic swallowing disorders.)

Head/Neck Cancer

No numerical data substantiate the incidence or prevalence of dysphagia following treatment for cancer involving the structures of the jaw, mouth, pharynx, larynx, and neck, although it is well known that this group of patients is prone to dysphagia. Dysphagia can be secondary to the removal of tissue, with subsequent sensory and motor loss, and to the effects of **radiation therapy** and **chemotherapy.** It is presumed that patients with significant tumor removal (more than 50% of the structure), or those with large tumors that are treated with radiation alone, have the highest risk for developing dysphagia. Evidence suggests that patients with pharyngeal resections and those with tumors involving the tongue base are more likely to suffer from dysphagia.

Head Injury

Dysphagia following severe head injury is common, although numerical data have not been reported. The secondary effects of head injury on cortical and respiratory function often preclude attempts at oral **alimentation.** Patients who are in semicomatose states are not able to concentrate or cooperate during attempts at eating. Problems with judgment make them unsafe candidates for feeding trials. In the acute setting, patients may be on ventilators or have **tracheostomy tubes** that interfere with their swallowing ability.

Prevalence data are available for patients who survive head injury and enter a **rehabilitation setting.** Lazarus and Logemann found that, in a mixed (type of injury and time after onset) group, approximately 50% of the patients they examined with videofluoroscopy had dysphagia. In those admitted to the head injury rehabilitation program during a 9-month period, 45% showed signs of dysphagia requiring further evaluation. Of those head-injured patients entering a rehabilitation setting, Winstein found that 33% were dysphagic on admission and that only 6% were dysphagic after 5 months of rehabilitation.

Progressive Neurologic Disease

Progressive neurologic diseases that commonly give rise to dysphagia include **Parkinson's disease** and its variants; **amyotrophic lateral sclerosis (ALS); multiple sclerosis (MS); myasthenia gravis (MG);** and **systemic rheumatic diseases,** such as **dermatomyositis, polymyositis, rheumatoid arthritis (RA), scleroderma,** and **Sjögren's syndrome.** Systemic rheumatic disorders are rarer than Parkinson's disease or MS, but deserve consideration in a discussion of dysphagia and neurologic disease. Because of the progressive nature of these disease processes, one is never certain at what point in the disease's progression that dysphagic symptoms occur. For example, some patients complain of dysphagia as the initial symptom of the disease, whereas others may never complain of dysphagia. In general, however, as disease severity increases, so does dysphagia. Complications from dysphagia, particularly those that threaten pulmonary function, may lead to **aspiration pneumonia** and death.

Parkinson's Disease. Although dysphagia secondary to Parkinson's disease appears to be common, accurate measurements are restricted by poor descriptions of the disease stage. However, most authors agree that dysphagia occurs in at least 50% of those with Parkinson's disease. The prevalence of dysphagia may be higher in those patients with Parkinson's disease who also have significant dementia.

Amyotropic Lateral Sclerosis. When ALS affects the **bulbar musculature**, dysphagia may be one of the first symptoms of the disease. Caroscio, Mulvihill, and Sterling found that of all patients with diagnosed ALS, 25% had bulbar-related symptoms at onset. Because not all patients with ALS develop specific bulbar signs, it is difficult to make a precise estimate of the prevalence of dysphagia. There are characteristics of disease progression affecting the bulbar musculature that typically result in dysphagia.

Multiple Sclerosis. Hartelius and Svensson found that in a large series of patients with MS, more than 33% had either chewing or swallowing problems. Similar to ALS, not all patients with MS are dysphagic, unless the bulbar musculature is involved. Because of the disease's tendency to produce ataxic symptoms, the incoordination between deglutition and breathing may predispose these patients to dysphagia, as well as to oral and pharyngeal muscle weakness and incoordination.

Myasthenia Gravis. In selected populations of patients with MG, approximately one third are dysphagic. The prevalence of dysphagia largely depends on the extent of muscle fatigue.

Polymyositis/Dermatomyositis. The prevalence of dysphagia after the diagnosis of either polymyositis or dermatomyositis is not known. As with other progressive neurologic conditions, their course and response to medical therapy may differ. Therefore the presence of dysphagia is variable. Because these diagnoses tend to involve the **proximal muscles**, swallowing can be affected.

Rheumatoid Arthritis. Geterude, Bake, and Bjelle found that 8 of 29 patients with RA had complaints of dysphagia. In a series of 31 patients with dysphagia and RA, Ekberg, Redlund-Johnell, and Sjoblom documented pharyngeal dysfunction in 20.

Scleroderma. As many as 90% of patients with scleroderma have complaints related to swallowing. Complaints usually are confined to the esophagus, although secondary effects on the oral and pharyngeal stages are known.

Sjögren's Syndrome. As many as 75% of patients diagnosed with Sjögren's syndrome have dysphagia. The potential of this syndrome to involve all stages of swallowing function is well known.

LEVELS OF CARE

The prevalence, etiology, and type of swallowing disorder that one might encounter depend in part on the setting in which the patient is seen. Traditionally, levels of care are divided into five categories: **acute, subacute, rehabilitation**, long-term care, and **home health.**

Acute Care Setting

In a survey of two acute care hospitals, Groher and Bukatman found the prevalence of swallowing-related disorders to be 13%. Most of these patients were in the intensive care units and the neurology and neurosurgery units. Because of the acute nature of their illnesses, patients in this setting often have multiple medical complications, require ventilators and tracheostomy tubes, require feeding tubes for nutrition, and have frequent changes in mental status. Because their stay in the hospital may be short (2 to 5 days), their swallowing needs must be addressed rapidly. Often there is not sufficient time (or patient cooperation because of changes in mental status) to order sophisticated laboratory tests. In this circumstance, the clinician must rely on the history of the patient and clinical evaluation to make a diagnosis and establish a treatment plan. If the patient is able to cooperate with laboratory testing and is a candidate for further rehabilitation, his or her future care is facilitated if the acute care clinician can document the swallowing disorder with an instrumental technique such as videofluoroscopy or **endoscopy.**

Subacute Care Setting

Patients admitted to the subacute care unit usually are not ready for a strenuous rehabilitation program. They may require additional medical monitoring, but not the type of costly care necessary for patients admitted to the acute care unit. If a swallowing treatment goal has been formulated in the acute setting, the action plan to achieve that goal is implemented in the subacute unit. For instance, if the goal is to wean the patient from his or her tracheostomy tube as a way to ensure swallowing safety, the swallowing team works toward that goal. If a patient continues to require tube feeding after leaving the acute care unit, a goal of the swallowing team in the subacute unit might be to begin restoring oral alimentation. Patients may stay in the subacute unit from 5 to 28 days. Following this admission, they may be discharged home, to a rehabilitation facility, or to a skilled nursing facility.

Rehabilitation Setting

Patients who enter rehabilitation settings usually are judged to have the physical stamina needed to complete a full day of tasks oriented toward restoring lost function. In most cases, the patient also is able to learn new information. Those with swallowing impairment may need to learn, or solidify their learning of, new swallowing strategies. The role of the speech-language pathologist is to teach the patient swallowing strategies (see Chapter 10). This may include special maneuvers or postures. It also may entail ordering specialized diets.

Commonly, the goal in the rehabilitation setting, as it pertains to swallowing, is to return the patient to a dietary level that is as near to normal as possible, while ensuring swallowing safety. Swallowing safety might be defined as the maintenance of nutrition and **hydration** without medical complications. Not only is it medically unsafe for a patient to draw food or fluid into the lungs, it is also unsafe not to maintain nutrition and hydration sufficient for normal bodily functions. For instance, lack of proper nutrition and hydration can lead to excessive fatigue, mental status changes, poor wound healing, **anorexia,** and a greater chance of developing infections. After 1 month of successful rehabilitation, the patient usually is discharged home. Those who develop medical complications during rehabilitation or who fail to improve to a level of partial independence may be discharged to a skilled nursing facility.

Long-Term Care Setting. Patients who enter long-term care facilities usually have failed rehabilitation, are not candidates for rehabilitation following acute hospitalization, are too ill to be at home, or have chronic medical conditions that require monitoring in a structured environment. The prevalence of swallowing disorders in this setting has been reported to be between 50% and 66%. The prevalence in this setting is high because the patients admitted to nursing home care settings have multiple medical problems that predispose them to dysphagia. For example, most are suffering from a neurologic disease that has compromised the swallowing musculature or has interfered with the cortical controls needed to complete the swallowing sequence. Their swallowing disorders are chronic. Some patients have experienced some recovery in their dysphagia, whereas others continue to rely on tube feedings. Those who have to rely on tube feedings after their hospital stay require reevaluation for the possibility of returning to oral feeding. For some, returning to oral alimentation is not possible. Because of the potential for patients in this setting to be medically fragile, it is easy for a slight change in medical status to decompensate their swallowing skills, rather than a new, major event such as stroke. An example of this phenomenon is a patient who is not swallowing a sufficient amount of liquids and then develops a urinary tract infection that results in a fever with generalized fatigue, anorexia, and a disinterest in eating. In this situation, the patient may not be ingesting enough calories to be able to sustain the strength needed to produce a safe swallow throughout the entire meal. Because of fatigue, these patients are more likely to evidence signs of dysphagia. Another example is a patient who has been eating well, but whose medications were changed. The unwanted side effect from that medication change could negatively affect the nervous system to create a problem with motor movement, and swallowing is secondarily affected. For example, medications that create sedative effects are capable of decompensating an already fragile swallow by slowing motor movement and by interfering with the cortical controls necessary to complete an entire meal. The potential for fluctuations in metabolism in this patient population often makes it difficult to establish a single factor that precipitated the dysphagia.

It is known that patients who are in long-term care facilities usually are in older age-groups. Not only do they suffer from the effects of diseases commonly found in older persons that result in dysphagia (e.g., stroke, Parkinson's disease), they also have impairments in swallowing as a result of the aging process. Changes in taste perception and in the strength and speed of the swallowing muscles are examples of changes resulting from the aging process. In a survey of more than 500 men and women between the ages of 50 and 79 years and living at home, Lindgren and Janzon found that 35% complained of dysphagia. This suggests that a large number of older persons may be at significant risk for dysphagic symptoms even when they are in reportedly good health.

The speech-language pathologist working in the skilled nursing facility is kept busy managing the large number of patients with swallowing disorders. Many patients with dysphagia are able to eat safely only if they are at the proper dietary level, and only if they are following the recommended feeding strategies. Any change in baseline metabolism or any new neurologic insult may decompensate their swallowing skills, so they are at risk for developing medical complications. Many times, the focus of therapeutic effort for the speech-language pathologist working in the skilled nursing facility is prevention of dysphagia by attempting to keep patients as safe as possible while eating, even in the circumstance of suspected dysphagia. Such preventive efforts may require direct intervention with behavioral and dietary treatment strategies, and entail monitoring of mealtime activities to ensure that patients who are at aspiration risk are following the prescribed dysphagia treatment plan.

Often, the mental or physical status of patients in the skilled nursing environment interferes with their ability to cooperate with a formal dysphagia evaluation. Clinicians have to rely on a combination of the medical history and detailed observations of each meal to set the treatment plan. If the patient is not eating orally, the clinician often must rely on the physical examination and on his or her judgment of how well the patient performs attempts at oral ingestion as part of that examination.

The chronic medical conditions of patients in long-term care facilities often are life threatening. For this reason, patients and their families may execute an Advance Directive (see Chapter 11). The Advance Directive is a statement by the patient (or family) of his or her desires and wishes regarding medical care in life-threatening situations, such as whether or not the patient wants to be resuscitated from cardiac arrest. Part of this directive may pertain to wishes regarding sustaining nutrition, especially when the support for nutrition may involve feeding tubes. Patients may elect to not be fed by a feeding tube despite the risk that they may aspirate and develop life-threatening pneumonia. In these cases, the role of the swallowing clinician is to recommend the safest mode of ingestion, ensuring that the patient and family understand the potential risks.

Home Health Setting. Patients who have left the hospital or the rehabilitation setting to go home may require additional monitoring or direct treatment from a therapist who performs his or her responsibilities in the patient's home environment. Patients who are unable to swallow should receive regular reevaluations of attempts at oral feeding, unless oral feeding is contraindicated by the medical care team. Most often, the clinician responsible for managing the swallowing disorder in the home environment is ensuring that the patient is following the swallowing strategies or has improved to a point at which consideration should be given to changing the dietary level. These changes often are made in consultation with the patient and family and are based on the physical examination and observations of eating.

THE SWALLOWING TEAM

The treatment of patients who have disruptions in swallowing can potentially involve many members of the medical community. Those who complain of dysphagia related to the head and neck may see an otolaryngologist, dentist, speech-language pathologist, or neurologist. To further define the disorder, these specialists often need the services of the radiologist. Patients who complain of a swallowing disorder that may be of esophageal origin may require the services of a gastroenterologist. If the swallowing disorder is related to an acute respiratory condition, these patients may be under the care of the pulmonologist, the pulmonary physical therapist, and the respiratory therapist. If the swallowing disorder is related to the process of feeding, the occupational therapist commonly is involved. If the swallowing disorder results in a compromised nutritional system, the dietitian is consulted. While the patient is in the hospital, the nurse often is involved in the identification and treatment of the swallowing disorder. In short, patients with swallowing disorders require the attention of many disciplines working in concert to achieve nutritional safety.

Ideally, health care professionals who are concerned about the patient's swallowing and nutritional safety work together toward the mutual goal of improving the patient's swallowing performance. Coordination of effort is important if timely results are to be achieved. Some medical centers have designated swallowing teams and swallowing team leaders. In many hospitals, the speech-language pathologist assumes the role of swallowing team leader. The role that each specialist on the team plays varies across settings. For instance, some gastroenterologists diagnose and treat swallowing problems that involve the esophagus, although disorders of the esophagus are not their specialty. Specific interest in the patient with a swallowing impairment also varies. For example, few radiologists have a specific interest in patients who complain of dysphagia. Because of this variance in interest and focus, not all swallowing disorder teams are the same, and in some cases, not all potential members are represented.

Speech-Language Pathologist

Speech-language pathologists have taken a leading role in the management of patients with dysphagia secondary to poor oral and pharyngeal swallowing mechanics. In most centers, they coordinate the swallowing team and are often the first professional to perform a history and physical examination specific to dysphagia. Based on the data gathered, they consult other members of the swallowing team, get approval from the patient's attending physician for any additional testing or referrals, and integrate the nonmedical and nonsurgical aspects of the dysphagia treatment program.

Otolaryngologist

Otolaryngologists are skilled in the evaluation of the upper digestive tract. In particular, their use of endoscopy for direct visualization of the structures of

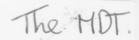

the nasopharynx, oropharynx, pharynx, and larynx adds information relative to the structural, sensory, and motor aspects of the pharyngeal stage of swallowing. In patients with head and neck cancer requiring surgery, otolaryngologists provide the surgical and postsurgical management. In this regard, they must be sensitive not only to issues of cancer control, but also to the preservation of speech and swallowing functions. The otolaryngologist may be involved with the surgical placement and removal of a patient's tracheostomy tube. These tubes frequently interfere with swallowing.

Gastroenterologist

Gastroenterologists who participate on the swallowing disorders team have a special interest in the esophagus. Because primary esophageal disorders that precipitate dysphagia can have secondary effects on the pharyngeal and oral stages of swallowing, it is important to include the gastroenterologist in the evaluation of the patient who may appear to have complaints that relate only to the oral or pharyngeal stages of swallowing (see Chapter 3). The gastroenterologist is familiar with the management of **gastroesophageal reflux disease (GERD)**, or heartburn, a symptom that may be related to dysphagia. The gastroenterologist may use special sensors that measure the amount of acid content in the alimentary tract using a test called **24-hour pH monitoring.** The gastroenterologist may use **manometry** to measure esophageal motility or may prescribe medications to improve esophageal motility or to control GERD. The gastroenterologist is responsible for the nonsurgical placement of a feeding tube in the stomach, which is called a **percutaneous endoscopic gastrostomy (PEG).**

Radiologist

The radiologist who is a member of the swallowing disorders team often has a special interest in the gastrointestinal tract. Radiologists provide both dynamic (videofluorographic) and static **(plane films)** imaging of the aerodigestive tract and lung fields. These studies often provide the diagnostic information that guides swallowing treatment.

Neurologist

Because most patients have dysphagia as a result of neurologic disease, the neurologist has an important role in managing swallowing problems. It is critical that patients who have dysphagic complaints without a known cause be considered for evaluation by the neurologist. Some neurologic diseases that precipitate dysphagia can be treated with medication. Finding a cause also is important in providing the patient with an explanation for the dysphagia and in providing a prognosis for future complications.

Dentist

Patients with dysphagic symptoms may be identified first by a dentist during routine dental care. Of particular interest to dentists are any oral-stage manifestations of swallowing disorders, such as problems with chewing, bolus formation, or dental disorders such as **osteoradionecrosis,** that make swallowing painful. The dental prosthodontist is skilled at making appliances for the oral cavity to facilitate swallowing in patients who have had removal of the oral structures secondary to cancer.

Nurse

The nurse has 24-hour responsibility for monitoring the patient's swallowing problem. Monitoring the amount of intake and recording it in the medical record is an important role for the nurse. During mealtime, nurses often identify problems in patients who are not suspected of having dysphagia, and they also provide the cues necessary to use swallowing strategies to help the patients with identified dysphagia. Other responsibilities of the nurse include administering tube feedings, maintaining good oral hygiene of the patient, and assigning volunteers to assist selected patients at mealtime.

Dietitian

The dietitian assesses patients' nutritional and hydration needs and monitors the patient's response to those needs. Because dysphagia often affects a patient's nutrition and hydration status, and because poor nutrition and hydration affects a patient's overall medical stability, it is important to involve the dietitian in the plan of care for the patient with dysphagia. Because the dietitian frequently monitors mealtime activities, he or she may be the professional who initially detects a swallowing disorder. If specialized dysphagic diets are ordered for the patient, the dietitian is responsible for obtaining those diets from the kitchen. If a patient is unable to eat orally, the dietitian may recommend tube feeding. Guidelines for the amount and rate of tube feeding commonly are provided by the dietitian.

Occupational Therapist

The occupational therapist is skilled in retraining patients to self-feed. If patients are unable to feed themselves because of either weakness or incoordination, the occupational therapist needs to be involved in their care. Special adaptive feeding devices, such as a **plate guard** or built-up utensils for easier grasping, are ordered by the occupational therapist to assist the patient in achieving feeding independence.

Pulmonologist/Respiratory Therapist

Although pulmonologists may not be regular members of the swallowing team, their patients often have swallowing disorders that require management by the team. Patients with respiratory disorders that require tracheostomy and ventilatory support (respirators) often have accompanying swallowing difficulty. Work with the respiratory therapist and pulmonologist to improve pulmonary integrity is an important step toward **decannulation.** Removing the patient from respiratory support often is a prerequisite for improving the swallowing response.

TAKE HOME NOTES

- Dysphagia is a symptom of a disease, not a primary disease. It is characterized by a delay or misdirection of something swallowed.
- A feeding disorder usually refers to a disorder in the process of food transport.
- The prevalence of dysphagia is highest in patients with neurologic disease.

- Patients in acute care intensive care units and in long-term care facilities tend to be most at risk for dysphagia.
- There may not be a clear link between dysphagic symptoms and the primary medical diagnosis of patients who reside in long-term care facilities.
- Patients in long-term care facilities are medically fragile, and their swallowing response can be easily decompensated by fatigue or by an acute medical condition such as an infection.
- Aspiration of liquid and food is the consequence of those materials entering the airway below the level of the vocal folds.
- Aspiration of liquid or food may produce a lung infection known as aspiration pneumonia.
- Respiratory impairments such as those requiring a tracheostomy tube also interfere with swallowing.
- The speech-language pathologist often is the coordinator of the swallowing team, and therefore needs to have an understanding of each team member's perspective of the dysphagic patient.

CHAPTER TERMS

24-hour pH monitoring A timed measurement, by specialized sensors attached to a tube, of the amount of stomach acid in the alimentary system

acute care setting Short-term health care offered in a hospital or emergency department for an illness with severe or rapidly developing symptoms

alimentation Providing food or fluid

amyotrophic lateral sclerosis (ALS) A progressive degeneration of the moto-neurons of the spinal cord, medulla, and cortex

anorexia Loss of appetite

aspiration Swallowed material that has entered the trachea below the level of the true vocal folds

aspiration pneumonia Aspiration of swallowed materials, which results in a lung infection

bulbar musculature The muscles of the head and neck that are innervated by the lower part of the brainstem

chemotherapy Treatment of certain types of cancer by the use of intravenous medications

decannulation The removal of a tube, as in tracheostomy

dermatomyositis An inflammation of the skeletal muscle connective tissue, often associated with skin lesions

endoscopy Using a rigid or flexible scope with a light source to view the alimentary tract

gastroesophageal reflux disease (GERD) Excessive acid in the stomach that enters the esophagus, pharynx, or mouth and may be associated with dysphagia

home health setting Medical care that is provided by specialists visiting the patient's home

hydration Providing adequate amounts of fluid

manometry A test that measures the pressures in the alimentary tract associated with swallowing *multiple sclerosis* An autoimmune, progressive, inflammatory neurologic disease affecting all parts of the central nervous system

myasthenia gravis A progressive disease affecting muscle strength, resulting from a chemical imbalance at the neuromotor junction

osteoradionecrosis A breakdown in bone or connective tissue caused by the side effects of radiation therapy

Parkinson's disease A progressive neurologic disorder affecting movement that results from damage in the basal ganglia

percutaneous endoscopic gastrostomy (PEG) A feeding tube placed in the stomach through an endoscope

plane films Still radiographs of a particular part of the body taken at varying angles or planes

plate guard A metal barrier attached to the side of a plate so that food is not pushed off the edge

polymyositis An inflammation of the skeletal muscle connective tissue particularly affecting the proximal limbs, neck, and pharyngeal muscles

proximal muscles Muscles of the body that are closer to the midline

radiation therapy A controlled radiation beam directed at a specific part of the body, often as an attempt to cure cancer

rehabilitation setting A medical facility designed to teach patients how to adapt to or compensate for a disability

rheumatoid arthritis An inflammation of the body's joints

scleroderma A connective tissue disorder that often affects the body's smooth muscles such as the esophagus

silent aspiration Swallowed material that goes below the vocal folds that does not produce a cough reflex

Sjögren's syndrome A disease of the connective tissue that also affects the lacrimal glands

subacute care setting A level of health care that is not acute, but is more oriented toward rehabilitation

systemic rheumatic disease Inflammation in the joints and connective tissue throughout the entire body

tracheostomy tube A plastic tube placed through a surgical incision in the neck below the level of the vocal folds to help the patient breathe; it provides direct access to the lungs for suctioning

videofluoroscopy A moving radiograph of the mouth, pharynx, larynx, and cervical esophagus during swallowing

SUGGESTED READINGS

Bine JE, Frank EM, McDade HL: Dysphagia and dementia in subjects with Parkinson's disease, *Dysphagia* 10:160-164, 1995.

Caroscio JT, Mulvihill MN, Sterling R: Amyotrophic lateral sclerosis: its natural history, *Neurol Clin* 5:1-8, 1987.

Daniels SK et al: Aspiration in patients with acute stroke, *Arch Phys Med Rehabil* 79: 14, 1998.

Ekberg O, Redlund-Johnell I, Sjoblom KG: Pharyngeal function in patients with rheumatoid arthritis, *Acta Radiol* 28:35, 1987.

Field LH, Weiss CJ: Dysphagia with head injury, *Brain Inj* 3:19, 1989.

Fulp SR, Castell DO: Scleroderma esophagus, *Dysphagia* 5:101, 1990.

Geterude A, Bake B, Bjelle A: Swallowing problems in rheumatoid arthritis, *Acta Otolaryngol* 111:1153, 1991.

Gordon C, Langton-Hewer R, Wade DT: Dysphagia in acute stroke, *Br Med J* 295:411, 1987.

Grande L et al: Esophageal motor function in primary Sjögren's syndrome, *Am J Gastroenterol* 88:378, 1993.

Groher ME, Bukatman R: Prevalence of swallowing disorders in two teaching hospitals, *Dysphagia* 1:3, 1986.

Hamdy S et al: Organisation and reorganisation of human swallowing motor cortex: implications for recovery after stroke, *Clin Sci* 99:151, 2000.

Hartelius L, Svensson P: Speech and swallowing symptoms associated with Parkinson's disease and multiple sclerosis: a survey, *Folia Phoniatr Logop* 46:9, 1994.

Hillel AD, Miller RM: Bulbar amyotrophic lateral sclerosis: patterns of progression and clinical management, *Head Neck* 11:51, 1989.

Horner J, Massey EW, Brazer SR: Aspiration in bilateral stroke patients, *Neurology* 40:1686, 1990.

Kuhlemeier K: Epidemiology and dysphagia, *Dysphagia* 9:209, 1994.

Layne KA et al: Using the Fleming index of dysphagia to establish prevalence, *Dysphagia* 4:39, 1989.

Lazarus C, Logemann JA: Swallowing disorders in closed head trauma patients, *Arch Phys Med Rehabil* 68:79, 1987.

Lieberman AN et al: Dysphagia in Parkinson's disease, *Am J Gastroenterol* 74:157, 1980.

Lindgren S, Janzon L: Prevalence of swallowing complaints and clinical findings among 50-79-year-old men and women in an urban population, *Dysphagia* 6:187, 1991.

McConnel FM et al: Surgical variables affecting postoperative swallowing efficiency in oral cancer patients: a pilot study, *Laryngoscope* 104:87, 1994.

Murray JP: Deglutition in myasthenia gravis, *Br J Radiol* 35:43, 1962.

Siebens H et al: Correlates and consequences of eating dependency in institutionalized elderly, *J Am Geriatr Soc* 34:192, 1986.

Smithard DG et al: The natural history of dysphagia following a stroke, *Dysphagia* 12:188, 1997.

Tally NJ et al: Onset and disappearance of gastrointestinal symptoms and functional gastrointestinal disorders, *Am J Epidemiol* 136:165, 1992.

Veis SL, Logemann JA: Swallowing disorders in persons with cerebrovascular accident, *Arch Phys Med Rehabil* 66:372, 1985.

Winstein CJ: Neurogenic dysphagia: frequency, progression, and outcome in adults following head injury, *Phys Ther* 63:1992, 1983.

CHAPTER 2

The Normal Swallow

FOCUS QUESTIONS

1   What are the key anatomic structures involved in swallowing?
2   What groups of muscles participate in swallowing?
3   What are the peripheral and central neurologic controls for swallowing?
4   What are the key components in moving a bolus through the alimentary tract?
5   How would all the components of a swallow response be described, beginning with the oral preparatory stage and ending in the stomach?
6   What are some issues to consider when describing the normal swallow of a person older than 65 years?

OVERVIEW

Swallowing can be divided into four stages: oral/preparatory, oral, pharyngeal, and esophageal. The division of swallowing into four separate stages may be misleading, because each stage is interdependent. Swallowing is best understood if swallowing performance is thought of as one behavior with four components that must act in an integrated manner if swallow success is to be achieved. This perspective has four implications for swallowing management: (1) that the source (stage involved) of swallowing disability may not be totally apparent or easily understood (see Chapter 3), (2) that disruption in one stage may interfere with another stage, (3) that focused treatment on one stage may affect the competency of other stages, and (4) that a complete evaluation for the dysphagic condition should include an evaluation of each component stage. Traditionally, the oral/preparatory stage is thought to be more volitional than either the pharyngeal or the esophageal stages, because it can be altered easily if a person concentrates on its activities. For most people, each swallow is not brought to the conscious level. It often accompanies more volitional acts of conversation. Its volitional components are manifested most often when a person has to swallow a pill or an unfamiliar bolus. The pharyngeal and esophageal stages normally are depicted as more reflexive than the oral stage, although conscious alterations of pharyngeal function, as occurs in sword swallowing, are possible. That the act of swallowing does not qualify as a true reflex is exemplified by the fact that its physiology changes depending on variations in the stimulus, such as different textures and volumes. This concept has led investigators to conclude that swallowing is best understood as a combination of preprogrammed events with neural circuitry that can adapt to change if needed. In this context, swallowing is viewed not as a true reflex, but as a programmed response to sensory stimuli.

ANATOMY

The anatomy of the upper aerodigestive tract as it pertains to swallowing is best understood in the lateral plane as illustrated in Figure 2-1. Grossly, the structures can be seen at rest: the jaw and lips anteriorly, the tongue and its relationship to the pharyngeal palate (velum) and nasopharynx, the spinal column and its relationship to the pharynx anteriorly, the vallecular space at the tongue base, the entrance to the airway **(laryngeal aditus)** and its relationship to the epiglottis and pharynx, the region of the **cricopharyngeal muscle** and its relationship to the spinal column, and the closed esophagus. Anatomic demarcations by region are seen in Figure 2-2. Anatomic landmarks mentioned in this section also can be appreciated by viewing dynamic radiographic and endoscopic images that delineate the anatomy of swallowing, as seen in the videotape that accompanies this text.

Oral/Preparatory Stage

Food boluses that require mastication are prepared in the oral cavity before the beginning of the swallow response. The tongue moves the bolus laterally to the molar ridges. Crushing, repetitive movements of the jaw reduce the bolus size. Once initiated, chewing continues reflexively, but can be altered by cortical inputs. Of course, this activity is not required for a liquid bolus;

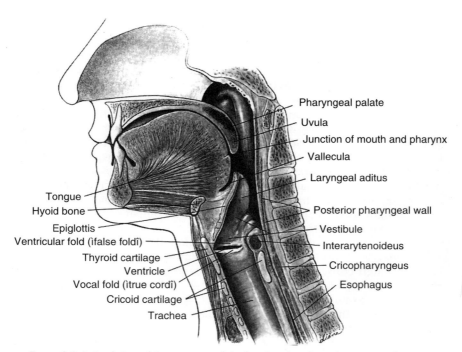

FIGURE 2-1 Lateral view of the anatomy of the head and neck pertinent to swallowing. (From Bosma JF et al: *Dysphagia* 1:24, 1986.)

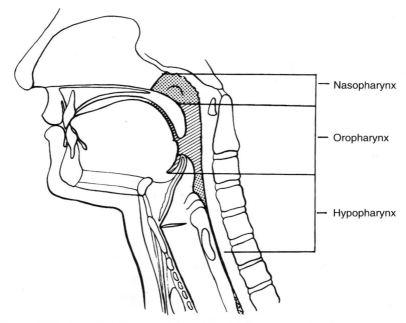

FIGURE 2-2 Lateral view of the anatomy of the head and neck with demarcations of three major regions: nasopharynx, oropharynx, and hypopharynx.

however, momentary containment by the tongue may be necessary so that the liquid bolus does not prematurely enter the airway. The temporalis, masseter, buccinator, and pterygoid muscles are the paired muscles that are active during solid-food preparation. This chewing activity stimulates the saliva glands, allowing moisture to form and lubricate the bolus for swallowing ease. Adequate saliva also is important to maintain good oral health (dentition), taste facilitation, and a normal acid-base balance in the stomach, particularly at night. The parotid, submandibular, and sublingual glands serve as the main conduits for saliva production. Their stimulation is accomplished through motor **autonomic fibers** carried by cranial nerves (CN) VII (facial) and IX (glossopharyngeal). The oral cavity is particularly rich in mechanical (touch, pressure) receptors on the tongue, teeth, gums, and palate. Sensory information from these mechanical receptors is transmitted via CN V (trigeminal) to the brainstem centers that coordinate swallowing efforts (see subsequent section, Neurologic Control of Swallowing). Other receptors that are sensitive to change in temperature also are carried by the sensory branch of CN V. Sensory information pertaining to taste (chemoreceptors) is mediated partially by CN VII on the anterior two thirds of the tongue and by CN IX on the posterior tongue. Sensory information pertaining to taste, temperature, and mastication is sent to the brainstem and is integrated in the **nucleus tractus solitarius (NTS)** of the medulla. Because it is known that a person can change his or her swallowing pattern volitionally (particularly during the oral/preparatory stage), it is assumed that higher cortical centers that modulate swallowing must exist. These higher centers undoubtedly are capable of exerting influence on the more programmed swallowing circuitry of the brainstem (e.g., by thinking about initiating or terminating a swallow).

Oral Stage

The oral stage of swallow begins after the bolus is prepared for swallowing. At the moment of the swallow response, the bolus is propelled into the oropharynx and then into the hypopharynx (see Figure 2-2). The key structure in this effort is the tongue. Before swallow, the tongue (CN XII, hypoglossal) cradles the bolus, pressing its edges against the hard palate as the swallow begins. When contracted at the moment of swallow, the extrinsic tongue muscles, primarily the digastric (CN V), mylohyoid (CN V), and geniohyoid (CN XII) muscles, allow the tongue to propel the bolus posteriorly. Through their connections to the hyoid bone, the hyoid bone is elevated in a superior and anterior plane. The posterior tongue is elevated by actions of the palatoglossus

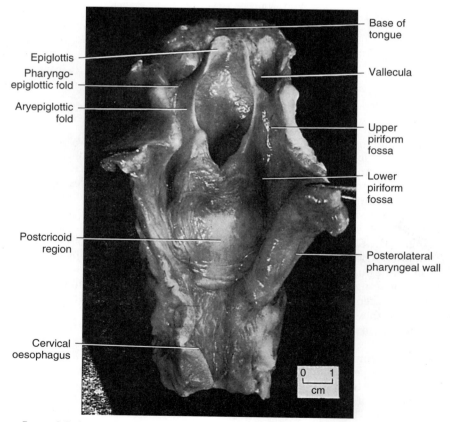

Epiglottis

Pharyngo-epiglottic fold

Aryepiglottic fold

Postcricoid region

Cervical oesophagus

Base of tongue

Vallecula

Upper piriform fossa

Lower piriform fossa

Posterolateral pharyngeal wall

0   1
cm

FIGURE 2-3 Anatomic specimen of the pharyngeal compartment as it surrounds the airway. The bolus flows into the vallecular spaces, around the epiglottis inferiorly into the piriform fossa before entering the esophagus.

muscle (CN X, vagus). The elevation of the velum to seal the nasopharynx is accomplished collectively by the palatopharyngeal muscle (CN X and XI) and the levator muscle of velum palatinum (CN X and XI). Although not technically part of the anatomy of the oral cavity and nasopharynx, the activity of airway closure (laryngotracheal protection) is physiologically linked with the onset of the oral stage of swallow. Key structures of airway closure include both the true and the false vocal folds (CN X, recurrent branch). Mechanical, chemical, and water-respondent receptors are abundant in this area. Sensation from these receptors is carried by the sensory branch (superior laryngeal nerve) of CN X.

Pharyngeal Stage

The major anatomic landmarks of the pharyngeal stage of swallow include the epiglottis, vallecular and piriform sinus spaces, thyroid and cricoid cartilages, larynx, cervical spine, and posterior pharyngeal wall (see Figures 2-1 and 2-3). The major muscles involved in propelling the bolus include the palatopharyngeal (CN X and XI) and stylopharyngeus (CN IX) muscles, which act to elevate and shorten the pharynx as the bolus arrives, and the superior (CN X and XI), medial (CN X), and inferior (CN X and XI) constrictor muscles. The inferior constrictor muscle comprises the oblique musculature of the thyropharyngeal muscle and the circular fibers of the cricopharyngeal muscle (Figure 2-4). Together with the circular and longitudinal musculature of the upper third of the esophagus, this makes up the functional unit called the **pharyngoesophageal segment (PES).** Gastroenterologists refer to this region

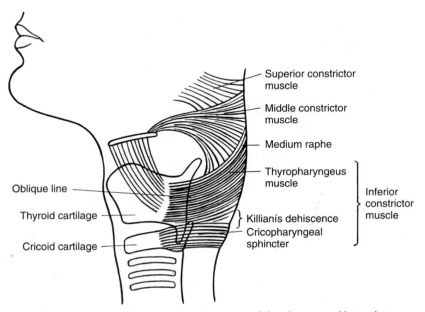

FIGURE 2-4 Lateral view of the major muscle groups of the pharynx and hypopharynx. The oblique fibers of the thyropharyngeus meet the circular fibers of the cricopharyngeal muscle. Together they form the inferior constrictor muscle.

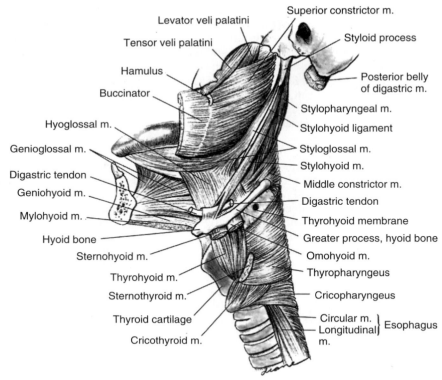

Figure 2-5 Lateral view of the key muscles of the head and neck used in swallowing. (From Bosma JF et al: *Dysphagia* 1:25, 1986.)

as the **upper esophageal sphincter (UES).** The PES remains closed during nonswallow moments by innervation from the sympathetic chain of the superior cervical ganglia. Relaxation is accomplished by parasympathetic signals (CN IX and X) sent to the brain during swallowing, belching, or retching. The course and relationship of the major muscles involved in swallowing during the oral/preparatory, oral, and pharyngeal stages of swallowing are illustrated in Figure 2-5.

Esophageal Stage

The esophagus is a closed muscular tube at rest that extends approximately 18 to 22 cm from the cervical (more proximal) portion (inferior to the hypopharynx) to its **distal** extension at the level of the stomach. It courses through the chest ventral to the lungs and around the aorta of the heart. It enters the stomach through the **diaphragmatic hiatus** (Figure 2-6). The upper third of the esophagus is composed of **striated muscle** that is under the control of the central nervous system (**nucleus ambiguus [NA], CN X**). The remaining two thirds is composed of **smooth muscle** controlled by autonomic nervous fibers that are integrated in the **dorsal motor nucleus** of CN X. The muscular

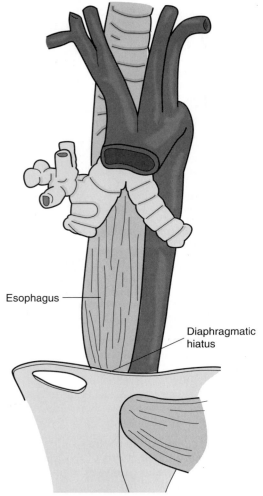

FIGURE 2-6 The esophagus courses through the chest cavity and through a hiatus in the diaphragm, ending at the level of the stomach.

Esophagus

Diaphragmatic hiatus

components at the superior end of the esophagus may be called the UES or PES, whereas those at the lower end are called the **lower esophageal sphincter (LES).** The multiple roles of the cranial nerves involved in swallowing are summarized in Table 2-1.

PHYSIOLOGY OF SWALLOWING

The physiology of swallowing is complex. Multiple groups of muscles innervated by **somatic** and **visceral** fibers are coordinated by a group of interneurons

Table 2-1	*Summary of Cranial Nerve Participation in Swallowing*	
CRANIAL NERVE	**CENTRAL NERVOUS SYSTEM**	**AUTONOMIC NERVOUS SYSTEM**
Trigeminal (V)	*Sensory:* Touch, pressure in mouth *Motor:* Muscles of mastification, tensor of velum palatinum, mylohyoid, digastric	None
Facial (VII)	*Sensory:* Taste, anterior tongue *Motor:* Lip muscles	*Visceral motor:* Sublingual, submandibular glands
Glossopharyngeal (IX)	*Sensory:* Taste, posterior tongue *Motor:* Stylopharyngeus, PES (parasympathetic fibers)	*Visceral motor:* Parotid gland
Vagus (X)	*Sensory:* Sensation from larynx, pharynx, trachea, esophagus *Motor:* Larynx and pharynx	*Visceral motor:* Smooth muscle of abdominal viscera
Accessory (XI) (cranial portion)	*Motor:* Same contributions as CN X, except for palatoglossus	
Hypoglossal (XII)	*Motor:* Intrinsic tongue muscles and extrinsic, except for mylohyoid and anterior digastric, muscles	

located in the medulla of the brainstem in the swallowing center. The normal swallow depends on the coordinated efforts of the four phases of swallowing. Rapid transport of the prepared bolus through the pharynx and into the stomach is a prerequisite for normal swallowing.

Bolus Movement

Normal swallowing performance depends on the rapid transfer of the bolus from the oral cavity to the stomach. A liquid bolus may pass through the pharynx within 2 seconds and enter the stomach in less than 5 seconds. Efficient movement is accomplished by the strength of the neuromuscular contraction exerted on the bolus and on the forces of gravity. Efficient bolus movement is accomplished when coordinated neuromuscular contractions and relaxations create zones of high pressure on the bolus and zones of negative pressure below the level of the bolus. Some parts of the swallowing chain, such as the esophagus, remain under negative pressure because of their location. Creating zones of high and low pressure is largely accomplished by the coordination and strength of the swallowing valves: lips, velum, airway closure, PES opening and closing, and LES opening and closing (Table 2-2). A person can experience

Table 2-2	*Swallowing Valves Important in Bolus Transport*
VALUE	FUNCTIONS
Lips	Closure builds intraoral pressure
Velum	Seals nasopharynx from foreign bodies
True vocal folds	Provide airway protection
False vocal folds	Provide airway portection
Pharyngoesopohageal	Relaxes for bolus entry, closes to avoid regurgitation
Lower esophageal sphincter	Relaxes for bolus entry, closes to avoid reflux

the difference in swallowing efficiency when trying to accomplish a swallow with the lips apart (valve open) compared with when they are closed. The tongue provides the initial positive driving force. The tongue's posterior deflection provides the basis for laryngeal elevation by applying traction to the hyoid bone. Efficient (i.e., timely and strong) laryngeal elevation helps create a negative zone of pressure in the pharynx, allowing the bolus to move rapidly, and therefore safely, from a zone of high pressure into a zone of negative pressure. Moving from a zone of high pressure into another zone of high pressure caused by a pathologic condition (e.g., muscle weakness or inco-ordination) inhibits bolus flow and results in **stasis** and residue that may be aspirated into the airway.

Swallowing Mechanics

After the bolus is prepared for swallowing, a number of physiologic events occur within a half second as the oral stage begins its transfer of the bolus to the pharynx. First, the true vocal folds adduct, followed closely by the movement of the tongue that sets the hyoid bone into motion. The lips are closed. This is followed by closure of the false vocal folds and then by opening of the PES. The final event in the swallow sequence is the reopening of the vocal folds and the resumption of tidal breathing (Figure 2-7).

As the tongue moves posteriorly (by contraction of the digastric, geniohyoid, and mylohyoid muscles), its base makes contact with the posterior pharyngeal wall that is moving anteriorly by the contraction and elevation of the oropharyngeal constrictor muscles. The posterior retraction of the tongue lifts the hyoid bone in a superior and anterior plane to the level of the mandibular ridge. Hyoid elevation is maintained throughout a large portion of the swallow (see Figure 2-7). Coupled with the closure of the nasopharynx by the velum, positive force is maintained on the bolus. By the tongue's connections to the hyoid bone, and the hyoid bone's connections to the thyroid and cricoid cartilages, the larynx is pulled up and forward, resting under the tongue base that now partially covers the opening to the airway. As the larynx rises, the cartilaginous epiglottis makes its descent over the top of the airway, completing an elaborate system of airway protection that allows the bolus to be directed toward the esophagus, rather than into the trachea. Rapid and complete laryngeal elevation (averaging approximately 2 to 3 cm) aids in

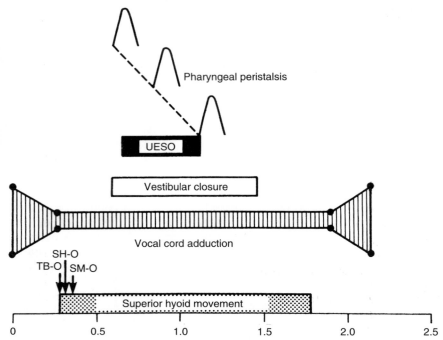

FIGURE 2-7 The relationship of the time of vocal fold closure and hyoid bone elevation during a 5-mL barium swallow. Bolus transit through the pharynx and across the upper esophageal sphincter (*UES*) begins and ends while the vocal folds are at maximal adduction. *SH-O,* Onset of superior hyoid movement; *SM-O,* onset of submental myoelectrical activity; *TB-O* onset of tongue base movement; *UESO,* UES opening. (From Shaker R et al: *Gastroenterology* 98:1482, 1990.)

creating negative pressure in the region of the hypopharynx. As the bolus enters the pharynx, it is divided by the **vallecular spaces** at the level of the tongue base, helping deflect it away from the airway as an additional component of airway protection. The five mechanisms of airway protection are summarized in Table 2-3. Simultaneously, the pharyngeal constrictor muscles act to narrow and shorten the pharynx, keeping sufficient positive pressure on the bolus as it flows into zones of negative pressure. Interestingly, the duration of pharyngeal muscle constriction is not affected by bolus size. As the bolus continues toward the esophagus, it remains divided, flowing into the two paired **piriform sinuses** lateral to the larynx in the region of the hypopharynx. The two halves of the bolus are rejoined as they enter the esophagus through the PES.

The PES opens by three mechanisms: (1) central nervous system–mediated relaxation in response to pharyngeal contraction (CN IX and X); (2) mechanical traction applied by the elevation of the hyoid bone, pulling open the PES after relaxation; and (3) the downward, driving force of the bolus into the cervical esophagus. A schematic representation of the three mechanisms that interact

Table 2-3	*Mechanisms of Airway Protection During Swallowing*
MECHANISM	ACTION
Airway closure	True and false vocal folds adduct, laryngeal aditus narrows
Laryngeal elevation	Larynx raises and tilts under the base of tongue
Tongue base retraction	Posterior tongue action causes tongue base to deflect bolus away from the airway
Epiglottis inverts	Rising larynx and thyroepiglottic ligament contraction allow the epiglottis to fold over the laryngeal aditus
Vallecular spaces	Bolus is divided and channeled around the airway

to open the PES is presented in Figure 2-8. Experimental evidence shows that the mechanics of opening the PES are related to bolus size. First, the larger the bolus, the earlier the muscular activity in the PES occurs in relationship to the moment of swallow. Second, the larger the bolus, the longer the PES remains open.

As the bolus enters the cervical esophagus, many of the structures that were active during the oropharyngeal stages return to their rest position. Before the delivery of the bolus, the esophagus has remained closed. As the bolus enters the esophagus, the mechanism of **peristalsis** delivers the bolus from the

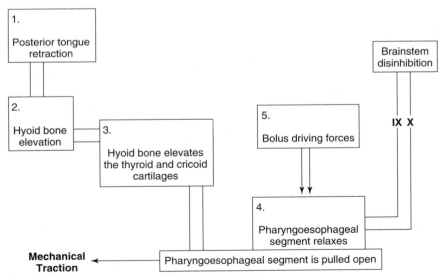

FIGURE 2-8 Schematic representation of the three mechanisms of pharyngoesophageal segment *(PES)* opening. They include mechanical traction *(1, 2, and 3)*, brainstem disinhibition *(4)*, and bolus driving forces *(5)*.

proximal esophagus to the distal esophagus and into the stomach. The first contractile wave of peristalsis usually is the strongest (Figure 2-9). Its strength depends on the efficiency of the pharynx to clear all of its contents. The more efficient the clearance, the stronger the wave. Peristalsis may be inhibited by multiple swallows of the same bolus. A secondary wave of activity to clear the esophagus of any residual is propagated by the bolus itself as it distends the esophagus on its path to the stomach. This is called the *secondary peristaltic wave.* The beginning of the peristaltic wave sends a message to the LES causing it to relax so that the bolus can flow into the stomach. Depending on the type of bolus (liquid versus solid), the speed of bolus transit may take from 3 to 10 seconds.

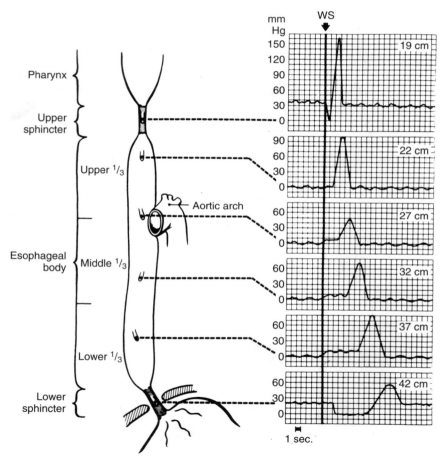

FIGURE 2-9 Manometric representation of esophageal peristalsis. Note that the first contractile wave is the strongest as the bolus first enters the esophagus. Note also that the pressure in the lower esophageal sphincter drops at the same time, with peak closure after the swallow has been completed.

NEUROLOGIC CONTROL OF SWALLOWING

Six cranial nerves provide the peripheral afferent and efferent component of the muscles involved in swallowing. In addition to their somatic component, visceral fibers are associated with the activity of the cranial nerves. The swallowing center in the medulla of the brainstem is the key integrator of swallowing performance. There are subcortical and cortical centers above the brainstem that, when stimulated, induce swallowing behavior; however, their specific role and connections to the swallowing center are not well understood.

Peripheral Controls

There are six key cranial nerves whose somatic and autonomic components are active in producing a normal swallow: CN V, VII, IX, X, the cranial portion of XI, and CN XII. CN V carries sensory (touch, pressure, and temperature) information from the oral cavity, and sends efferent fibers to the muscles of mastication. It also is the motor to the external hypoglossal muscles (digastric, mylohyoid) that aid in tongue retraction at the moment of swallow. CN VII is the motor to the facial muscles (lip control) and has a specialized sensory branch, the **chorda tympani,** that mediates taste. Motor autonomic fibers associated with CN VII from the **superior salivatory nucleus** of the brainstem provide moisture to the oral cavity through the submandibular and sublingual glands. The activity of chewing serves as the stimulus for this motor response. CN IX primarily has sensory functions (touch and temperature) in the oropharynx and is the primary carrier of taste on the posterior aspect of the tongue. Through communications with the **inferior salivatory nucleus** of the brainstem, autonomic motor fibers provide the majority of moisture to the oral cavity by way of the parotid gland. The motor responsibilities of CN IX are to the stylopharyngeus muscle and the PES in conjunction with CN X from the **pharyngeal plexus.**

CN X plays a key role in swallowing because of its extensive innervations into striated and smooth muscle, not only into the muscles used primarily for swallowing, but also into organs, such as the lungs, that may be related to normal swallowing performance because of their role in respiration. In the peripheral head and neck region, four main components of CN X relate directly to swallowing performance (Figure 2-10): (1) the pharyngeal branch, which combines with CN IX in the pharyngeal plexus to innervate the PES; (2) the superior laryngeal nerve, which provides sensory innervation to the epiglottis and to the structures in and around the airway; (3) the inferior or recurrent laryngeal nerve, which supplies most of the motor components to the muscles involved in airway closure and to the musculature in the region of the PES; and (4) the autonomic fibers of CN X that arise from the dorsal vagal nucleus in the brainstem, which innervate the smooth muscle portion of the esophagus, heart, and lungs. The cranial portion of CN XI runs concurrently with CN X in its innervation of the pharyngeal constrictor musculature.

The last cranial nerve to play a role in swallowing is CN XII. This cranial nerve is the motor to all of the intrinsic tongue musculature and to most of the extrinsic tongue muscles. A summary of the cranial nerves and their relationship to swallowing is presented in Table 2-1.

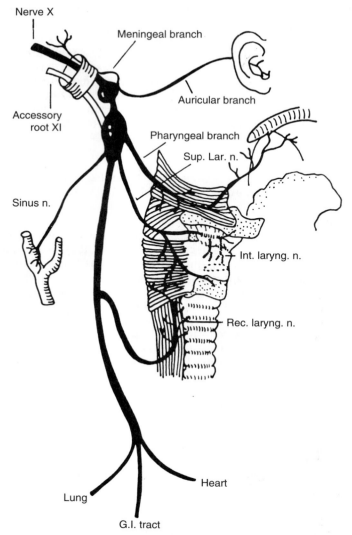

Figure 2-10 Schematic representation of the three peripheral branches of CN X: the pharyngeal branch to the region of the velum and pharynx; the internal and recurrent branches to the larynx; and the autonomic branch to the heart, lungs, and gastrointestinal tract.

Brainstem Controls

Two specialized nuclei located in the medullary portion of the brainstem are responsible for the integration of swallowing. The NTS integrates sensory information important to swallow (touch, temperature, and taste). It receives afferent input from CN V, VII, IX, and X. The NTS also receives sensory input from cardiovascular and respiratory brainstem nuclei, which are located near the swallowing center. These connections are important because respiration must cease during swallow. The NTS transfers sensory information to the motor output integrator, the NA. The NA then provides the motor output to the muscles of swallowing via CN V, VII, IX, X, XI, and XII. Visceral efferent fibers course with CN VII and IX to provide sufficient moisture to the oral cavity. The origin of these fibers, respectively, is from the superior and inferior salivatory nuclei located close to the NA. Fibers from the dorsal nucleus of CN X also course through the NA. Other specialized nuclei responsible for neurologic control of esophageal function are in close proximity to the NA. Because of the total integration of both sensory and motor information received from multiple sites and cranial nerves involved in swallowing, some authors refer to the NTS and NA collectively as the *swallowing center*. The anatomic relationship of the key brainstem nuclei involved in swallowing is presented in Figure 2-11.

Central Neurologic Controls

Axons from the NTS ascend to the pons and may be joined by sensory tracts outside the corticobulbar system, such as those from the hypothalamus. The hypothalamus has a role in regulating thirst and hunger responses. All ascending sensory information is carried through the thalamus to the sensorimotor strip of the parietal lobe. The anterolateral region immediately in front of the precentral cortex is thought to play a role in the motor aspects of swallowing at the cortical level, with descending motor tracts going through the region of the substantia nigra of the subcortex, to the reticular formation of the pons, with terminations in the swallowing center in the brainstem. Motor fibers from the hypothalamus, limbic forebrain, and cerebellum also may influence swallowing behaviors. Studies using magnetic resonance imaging techniques have identified multiple areas of activation in the cortex during swallowing,

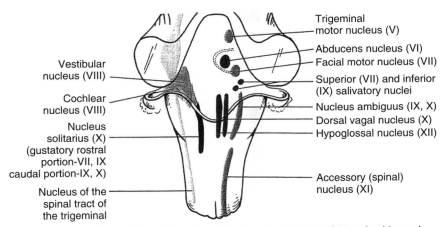

FIGURE 2-11 A view of the relationships of the key brainstem nuclei involved in swallowing. Most nuclei are within close proximity in the dorsal and ventral parts of the medulla.

including the precentral cortex, lateral postcentral gyrus, supplementary motor region, and anterior cingulate gyrus (see Chapter 4 for greater detail on cortical control mechanisms).

SWALLOWING AND AGING

Swallowing disorders usually are the result of neurologic impairment (see Chapter 4). Because neurologic disease is more common in older persons, it is important to have an understanding of how the aging process affects the swallowing response. This understanding is important because clinicians often have to separate the effects of disease on swallowing performance from the effects of normal aging. Further, clinicians must be able to assess the impact of age on the swallowing performance of a person with a neurologic disease that may be a contributor to a disruption in any part of the **alimentary tract.**

Physiologic Changes

Aging often results in reduced muscle mass and connective tissue elasticity. Loss of the integrity of muscle mass and elasticity results in a loss of strength and speed of movement. This may affect the muscles of the head and neck region, as well as the muscles of respiration. These changes affect an older person's swallow performance. Evidence suggests that the swallow of an older person is distinguished from a younger person by speed alone. Although a reduction in the speed of swallow may not cause dysphagia, it may put someone at greater risk for bolus misdirection. When neurologic disease or fatigue puts stress on these muscles, they may lack the necessary reserve to perform normally. In this context, the swallow of older persons may be normal but may be more easily decompensated.

Oral Stage. The tongue in an older person may undergo changes that affect normal function. Fatty tissue deposits in the tongue and its connecting fibers increase, which may result in a reduction in muscle strength and range of motion. These same changes can be found in the muscles of mastication. Robbins found that the ability of older persons to sustain isometric tasks involving the tongue is reduced, but that their ability to produce sufficient pressure generation for swallow is intact. The implication of Robbins' work is that, under conditions of stress (isometrics), swallowing performance may not be normal. Older persons also suffer from a loss of primary taste receptors, and some report a diminished sense of smell. Coupled with a loss of saliva, probably as a side effect of medical therapy, the sensory input system that is crucial to swallow performance may be at risk. Poor dentition may contribute to painful swallow **(odynophagia)** or to poor occlusal relationships that result in less efficient mastication. Difficulty in mastication and complaints of lack of taste ultimately result in poor oral intake and the prospect of **undernutrition.**

Pharyngeal Phase. Experimental studies have shown that the duration of airway closure may be reduced in older persons, although this may be more related to a reduction in respiratory capacity rather than in primary changes in vocal fold movement. Coupled with a reduction in the range of opening of the PES, older persons may be more likely to experience bolus residue that may enter the unprotected airway. Selley et al. demonstrated that the protective response of exhalation following a swallow is less common in older persons. Investigators who have made pressure measurements (manometry) within the PES have found that the pressures within the sphincter are lower in older persons. This implies that, in older persons, the barrier to **regurgitated** or **refluxed** contents from the esophagus may not be as efficient when compared with that of younger persons.

Esophageal Phase. Some experimental evidence suggests that the strength of esophageal peristalsis is compromised by the aging process. Although unproved, this may be more a function of the loss of strength in the striated proximal esophagus and its ability to provide an initial contraction strong enough to trigger a normal peristaltic response. Similar to the manometric findings in the PES, there is evidence that, in older persons, the LES pressure barrier to stomach contents may not be as strong as that in younger controls.

TAKE HOME NOTES

- Swallowing is accomplished by a complex interaction of striated and smooth muscles whose sensory and motor components are carried by multiple cranial nerves.
- The cranial nerves involved in swallowing send sensory information to the NTS. Motor components are organized in the NA. Together, the NTS and NA compose the swallowing center, which is located in the medulla of the brainstem.
- The preparation and movement of a bolus during swallowing theoretically can be conceived of as a series of valves that must open and close in a coordinated manner. This activity creates zones of high pressure around the bolus and zones of negative pressure below the level of the bolus. These pressure mismatches, together with gravity, create bolus flow.
- Respiration is arrested during swallowing. Protection of the airway to achieve a safe swallow is multifaceted. It is accomplished by primary airway closure at the level of the true and false vocal folds, laryngeal elevation, tongue base retraction, and epiglottic tilt.
- The process of aging does not create dysphagia, but may contribute to it, especially when a person is decompensated by disease.

CASE EXAMPLE

An 86-year-old man recently had heart surgery. After his surgery, he had a stroke affecting the premotor cortex of the left hemisphere. He has a history of depression treated with an antidepressant. He also had experienced Bell's palsy in the past, which affected CN VII in the upper and lower half of the left side of his face. He presented to the clinician with dysphagia. On examination, the patient complained that he was having difficulty chewing and that food did not taste good. He noted considerable choking and a feeling that food was sticking in his throat. Physical examination of cranial nerve function revealed weakened right facial musculature from the stroke and weakened left facial musculature from the prior Bell's palsy. He was unable to make a tight lip seal because of bilateral weakness in CN VII. His tongue deviated to the right upon protrusion, and range of motion was reduced (CN XII). Inspection of the oral cavity revealed moderate **xerostomia**. The patient's voice was hoarse and breathy, although the velum rose evenly when the gag reflex was tested. His swallowing study showed poor bolus preparation, limited laryngeal elevation, pharyngeal stasis on pudding textures, and aspiration of thin liquids at the moment of swallow. His clinician concluded that the patient's poor bolus preparation could have been secondary to multiple factors: tongue weakness, poor motor control from the involvement of a cortical motor area known to be important to bolus preparation, and lack of taste appreciation secondary to xerostomia (medication side effect) and to probable involvement of the chorda tympani branch of CN VII (on the left). It was further concluded that his pharyngeal symptoms were secondary to poor laryngeal elevation caused by tongue weakness. This resulted in a reduction in the opening of the PES, making it difficult for pudding to enter the esophagus, which caused him to feel as if food was sticking in his throat. Liquids were aspirated because the vocal folds could not close fast enough. This was a result of the involvement of the recurrent branch of CN X, which may have been damaged during the heart surgery, combined with the failure of the larynx to forcefully elevate and tilt forward because the tongue was weak. The pharyngeal branch of CN IX and X was unaffected, as evidenced by an intact gag reflex.

CHAPTER TERMS

alimentary tract Functionally defined as the system for getting nutrients into the body, including mouth, throat, esophagus, and stomach

autonomic fibers Fibers under control of the autonomic nervous system that assist in independent self-control of muscles (usually smooth) and glands

chorda tympani A specialized branch of CN VII that conveys taste sensation on the tongue and whose efferent fibers stimulate moisture from the submandibular and sublingual glands

cricopharyngeal muscle A circular band of muscle that sits between the cervical esophagus and the hypopharynx; remains closed, except during swallowing

diaphragmatic hiatus An opening in the diaphragm that allows the esophagus to connect to the stomach

distal Away from, or farthest from, the center

dorsal motor nucleus Nucleus in the brainstem mediating efferent input to internal organs, including the heart, lungs, and esophagus

inferior salivatory nucleus Located in the pons, it sends autonomic fibers to the parotid gland to provide moisture to the oral cavity

laryngeal aditus The top, or opening, into the larynx

lower esophageal sphincter (LES) Group of muscles at the distal end of the esophagus that relax during swallowing to allow contents to enter the stomach

***nucleus ambiguus* (NA)** Medullary nucleus that integrates the motor activities associated with swallowing

***nucleus tractus solitarius* (NTS)** Medullary nucleus that integrates the sensory activities associated with swallowing

odynophagia Painful swallowing

peristalsis Progressive, involuntary, wavelike movement, particularly common in the esophagus

pharyngeal plexus A network of nerves in the posterior pharyngeal wall that give rise to portions of CN IX and X

***pharyngoesophageal segment* (PES)** Functional region of swallowing composed of contributions of the thyropharyngeal and cricopharyngeal muscles of the hypopharynx and the oblique and circular muscles of the cervical esophagus

piriform sinuses Pyramidal spaces in the hypopharynx lateral to the larynx through which a bolus flows before entering the esophagus

reflux The return of stomach contents superiorly into the esophagus, throat, or mouth

regurgitation The return of undigested food from the esophagus into the throat or mouth

smooth muscle Muscle primarily under control of the autonomic nervous system

somatic Pertaining to striated muscle in the peripheral portion of the nervous system

stasis Stoppage of the normal flow of material

striated muscle Muscle under control of the central nervous system

superior salivatory nucleus A nucleus in the pons located dorsomedially to the facial nerve nucleus responsible for providing moisture to the oral cavity

undernutrition A subtype of malnutrition characterized by lack of sufficient nutrients to maintain normal bodily functions

***upper esophageal sphincter* (UES)** Most common term used by the gastroenterologist to refer to the opening to the esophagus

vallecular spaces Spaces lateral to the tongue base that divide a swallowed bolus, diverting it past the airway

visceral Generally pertaining to smooth muscle organs and glands

xerostomia Dryness, particularly in the oral cavity

SUGGESTED READINGS

Bass NH, Morell M: The neurology of swallowing. In Groher ME, editor: *Dysphagia: diagnosis and management,* Newton, Mass, 1997, Butterworth-Heinemann.

Castell JA et al: Effect of head position on the dynamics of the upper esophageal sphincter and pharynx, *Dysphagia* 8:1, 1993.

Cook IJ et al: Timing of videofluoroscopic, manometric events, and bolus transit during the oral and pharyngeal phases of swallowing, *Dysphagia* 4:8, 1989.

Donner MW, Bosma JF, Robertson DL: Anatomy and physiology of the pharynx, *Gastrointest Radiol* 10:196, 1985.

Jacob P et al: Upper esophageal sphincter opening and modulation during swallowing, *Gastroenterology* 97:1469, 1989.

Logemann JA et al: Closure mechanisms of laryngeal vestibule during swallowing, *Am J Physiol* 262:G338, 1992.

Martin RE, Sessle BJ: The role of the cerebral cortex in swallowing, *Dysphagia* 8: 195, 1993.

Martin RE et al: *Cerebral cortical representation of autonomic and voluntary swallowing in humans: a fMRI study*, Burlington, Vt, 1999, Dysphagia Research Society [Abstract].

Miller AJ: Swallowing: neurophysiologic control of the esophageal phase, *Dysphagia* 2:72, 1987.

Miller AJ: Neurophysiological basis of swallowing, *Dysphagia* 1:91, 1986.

Robbins J: Normal swallowing and aging, *Semin Neurol* 16:309, 1996.

Selley WG et al: Respiratory patterns associated with swallowing: part 2—neurologically impaired dysphagic patients, *Age Ageing* 18:173, 1989.

Tracy JF et al: Preliminary observations on the effects of age on oropharyngeal deglutition, *Dysphagia* 4:90, 1989.

C H A P T E R   3

Signs and Symptoms of Dysphagia

FOCUS QUESTIONS

1   What is the difference between a sign of a disorder and a symptom of a disorder?
2   What are the signs and symptoms of dysphagia?
3   How would the signs and symptoms associated with oropharyngeal impairment be distinguished from those associated with esophageal impairment?

Identification of a swallowing disorder enables medical specialists to provide the most efficacious diagnostic and treatment strategies. Early identification and treatment may help avoid adverse medical complications such as under-nutrition or respiratory infection. Because a variety of medical specialists can be involved in the care of the patient with dysphagia (see Chapter 1), all must be capable of detecting the signs and symptoms characteristic of dysphagia. Some signs may be overt, such as those in the patient who coughs while eating, whereas others may not be overt, such as those in the patient who may not have a swallowing complaint but comes to the swallowing specialist with a history of unexplained pneumonia. A radiographic evaluation of swallowing may reveal that food or fluid is silently entering the airway during swallow, resulting in aspiration-related pneumonia.

SYMPTOMS OF DYSPHAGIA

Symptoms usually are defined as any perceptible change in bodily function that the patient notices. This change eventually leads the patient to seek medical help when it causes pain or discomfort or negatively impacts his or her lifestyle. Some people have adverse medical symptoms and ignore them until the severity of their problem significantly affects their physiologic or mental health. Others seek immediate medical attention. Both groups may be diagnosed with a disorder that is similar in type and severity.

Patient Description

The physical examination of a patient with dysphagia may begin by asking him or her to describe the symptoms. Some common symptoms are detailed in Table 3-1. Because dysphagia often is secondary to neurologic disease that also may compromise communication skills, not all patients can provide a report of their symptoms. Because of cortical deficits, others may give unreliable or scant information. There is anecdotal evidence that many patients with dysphagia do not seek immediate medical attention; rather, they make changes in their eating habits to accommodate their symptoms, such as chewing food more finely or eliminating troublesome items from their menu. Others know that they are having difficulty swallowing but have a difficult time describing the specifics of their symptoms. Often it is difficult for them to remember how long those symptoms have been apparent. This may be due to the inherent flexibility of the swallowing tract to accommodate changes in function. Only when these accommodations no longer provide relief, or are too difficult to execute, does the patient seek medical attention. Some patients may have symptoms of dysphagia but ignore them. For example, one study performed on 56 older persons who were not complaining of dysphagia found that a large majority had radiographic abnormalities during swallowing tests. Such abnormalities included poor esophageal motility and pharyngeal weakness.

For patients who are able to communicate symptoms of their dysphagia, a detailed description may be useful in helping establish a diagnosis. Detailed descriptions also may be used to help the examiner focus on the types of diagnostic tests that may be most useful in delineating the source of the patient's complaint. The relationship between the accuracy of a patient's complaint and the final diagnosis has not been investigated extensively. Whether the complaint is useful in guiding the diagnostic process also has not been experimentally verified. Nonetheless, asking the patient to describe his or her problem is a common point of departure in the dysphagia examination.

Table 3-1 *Examples of Signs and Symptoms Associated with Dysphagia*

Symptom	Sign
Difficulty chewing	Food spills from lips; excessive mastication time of soft food; poor dentition; tongue, jaw, or lip weakness
Difficulty initiating swallow	Mouth dryness (xerostomia); lip or tongue weakness
Drooling	Lip or tongue weakness; infrequent swallows
Nasal regurgitation	Bolus enters or exits the nasal cavity as seen on radiographic swallowing study
Swallow delay	Radiographic study identifies transport beyond normal standard
Food sticking	Radiographic study identifies excessive residue in mouth, pharynx, or esophagus after completed swallow
Coughing and choking	Coughs on trial food attempts; material enters the airway on radiographic study
Coughing when not eating	Radiographic study shows aspiration of saliva or lung abnormality
Regurgitation	Undigested food in mouth; radiographic study shows food returning from esophagus to pharynx or mouth mucosal irritation on endoscopy; pH probe study positive for acid reflux
Weight loss	Unexplained weight loss; measurement of weight is below ideal standard

The literature suggests that patients who report dysphagic symptoms that can be localized to the esophageal region may be more useful than those who complain of disorders that may be pharyngeal or oral in their suspected origin. However, the level of esophageal involvement may not be easily localized. In one large study of patients who were found to have confirmed esophageal disease, most who pointed to the lower esophagus and had confirmed lower esophageal lesions were accurate. However, a significant number (30%) pointed to the upper neck and chest as the source of their discomfort. Other investigators have found that a significant number of patients who complained of food sticking at the level of the pharynx did have abnormalities at this level; however, the primary source of that abnormality often was found to be in the esophagus. This suggests that patients complaining of dysphagia localized to the neck and pharynx should have that specific region investigated, as well as undergo studies appropriate to the esophagus. One study found that if patients who complained of food sticking in the region of the neck also complained of respiratory symptoms (congestion, wheezing, and cough), the **sensitivity** of their dysphagia localized to the pharynx improves. Another group of investigators found that subtypes of esophageal disorders (**motility** versus **obstructive**) could be determined by patient report if the patient complained of a cluster of symptoms, such as heartburn with dysphagia, prior **dilation**, pain, and weight loss, rather than if he or she complained of heartburn alone. In general, studies agree that the complaint (dysphagic symptoms) presented by the patient correlates better with the findings when the problem after diagnosis is judged to be severe.

Some clinicians find it useful to explore a patient's dysphagic symptoms by questionnaire. A sample questionnaire is presented in Figure 3-1. This method may help ensure that all relevant questions relating to the patient's symptoms are addressed by the examiner. It also gives the patient a chance to think carefully about his or her symptoms before responding. No comparison between the standardized dysphagia questionnaire and the structured clinical interview as it relates to diagnostic approach or accuracy has been made. One recent study by Wallace, Middleton, and Cook sought to develop a symptom severity assessment tool. Their tool is a 19-point questionnaire designed to evaluate initial dysphagic symptom severity in comparison with dysphagic symptoms after therapy. Initial results indicted that their test was useful in documenting change in patients treated for Zenker's diverticulum. Their rationale for such a tool stems from the fact that a questionnaire method may be useful in documenting the effects of a swallowing intervention. In another study, the complaints of patients with head and neck cancer and oropharyngeal dysphagia were compared with their videofluorographic findings. The complaints and the videofluorographic results rarely correlated. Neither the site or severity of dysphagia could be determined from the patient's subjective report of the problem. A common finding was that the objective radiographic evidence showed a more severe problem than that reported by the patient.

Obstruction. One of the most common complaints from dysphagic patients is that food or fluids "get stuck." Most often, they report that the sticking sensation is in the throat or esophagus. Some patients do not use the word *stuck* but may use the word *fullness*. When they localize the feeling of obstruction to

1. Do you have difficulty chewing your food?   Yes   No

2. If so, which foods give you the most trouble? Underline any that apply.

    A. Solids (example: meats)

    B. Liquids (example: water)

    C. Semisolids (example: cottage cheese, applesauce, or cereal)

3. If you underlined a category in question number 2, list some of the:

    Specific solids:

    Specific liquids:

    Semisolids:

4. Do you have difficulty lining up your teeth?   Yes   No

5. Does food go all over your mouth, and is it
   difficult getting it together to swallow it?   Yes   No

6. Do you have trouble opening and closing your jaw?   Yes   No

7. Is the sensation in your mouth decreased?   Yes   No

8. Do you choke when eating?   Yes   No

9. If so, do you choke before you swallow, when
   you are chewing, or after you swallow?   Yes   No

10. Is it hard for you to:

    A. Lift your tongue?   Yes   No

    B. Move it from side to side?   Yes   No

    C. Move it from front to back?   Yes   No

11. Do you eat/drink more slowly now than before surgery? Yes   No

12. Do you eat/drink one category more slowly than others?

    Solids: Yes   No

    Liquids: Yes   No

    Semisolids: Yes   No

13. Does food catch in the:

    A. Left side of your throat?   Yes   No

    B. Right side of your throat?   Yes   No

    C. Left side of your mouth?   Yes   No

    D. Right side of your mouth?   Yes   No

    E. Behind your Adam's apple?   Yes   No

14. Do you need to pump your tongue many times
    to collect food to swallow?   Yes   No

15. Do you feel you have to swallow three or more
    times so all the food will go down?   Yes   No

16. Do you have trouble swallowing pills?   Yes   No

17. Do you cough up food?   Yes   No

18. If so, does the food come up:

    A. While chewing?   Yes   No

    B. After the food is swallowed?   Yes   No

Figure 3-1 Sample dysphagia questionnaire. (From Baker BM, Fraser AM, Baker CD: *Dysphagia* 6:11, 1991. © Springer-Verlag GmbH & Co. KG)

19. Do small amounts of food/liquids ever fall out
    of your mouth:

    A. Before you swallow?   Yes   No

    B. After you swallow?   Yes   No

20. Do you have a gurgly voice after you eat?   Yes   No

21. Do you feel the need to clear your throat after
    swallowing or eating a meal?   Yes   No

22. Do you have trouble controlling drooling?   Yes   No

23. Does food or liquid leak out of your:

    A. Trachea?   Yes   No   Not applicable

    B. Fistula?   Yes   No   Not applicable

24. Do you ever have to clean your mouth out after
    eating because food has become stuck?   Yes   No

25. Do you ever have to "wash down" your food
    with liquids?   Yes   No

26. Do you eat as much now as you did before
    your surgery?   Yes   No

27. Have you changed your diet in any way that is
    not mentioned above?   Yes   No

You are encouraged to add additional helpful information.

FIGURE 3-1 Cont'd.

the throat, they often describe their complaint as "a lump in the throat" when eating. The medical term for this feeling is *globus*. Some physicians have used the term *globus hystericus* to describe this sensation, because it was once thought that the description of a lump in the throat usually was associated not with **organicity**, but with symptoms of **hysteria**. Technically, the term *globus hystericus* is reserved for patients who complain of a lump in the throat that is relieved by swallowing or talking; it is not used to refer to a cause for dysphagia. However, use of the term *globus sensation* often is associated with the dysphagic person who complains that food is sticking at the level of the cervical esophagus. Although early investigators reported that they rarely found a cause for the globus sensation (i.e., patients were hysterical), recent reports suggest that with the appropriate battery of diagnostic tests, most patients who complain of globus are found to have an identifiable disease (see Chapter 6).

Liquids Versus Solids. Patients may report a change in their dietary habits that is associated with perceived dysphagia. For instance, those who complain of the globus sensation often have more difficulty swallowing solids than liquids. Classically, patients with solid-food dysphagia are more likely to have disorders of esophageal origin, whereas those who complain of dysphagia for liquids are more likely to have oropharyngeal dysphagia. However, this dichotomy may be artificial, because it is well known that persons with oropharyngeal dysphagia can have dysphagia for liquids and solids, and some forms of esophageal dysphagia evoke complaints regarding liquids and solids. When patients complain of choking on liquids or solids, a more pharyngeal-focused cause is suggested, whereas those who report dysphagia for liquids and solids without choking episodes may have a more esophageal-focused cause. Gastroenterologists who suspect the esophagus as the source of dysphagia may use a decision tree such as the one presented in Figure 3-2 to assist in diagnosis. Such a decision tree has not been validated against a large number of patients with confirmed diagnoses; however, the concept is useful because the symptoms related to the represented diseases are well known, and the number of potential causes for esophageal dysphagia is limited. Patients are asked questions that are related to diet (solids versus liquids), intermittent versus progressive symptoms, and the presence of heartburn. In general, patients with solid-food dysphagia are at risk only for more obstructive types of dysphagia in the esophagus. Patients who complain of dysphagia with both liquids and solids more commonly have disorders of esophageal motility. A decision tree for suspected oropharyngeal dysphagia has not been developed, primarily because of overlapping (and therefore nonspecific) symptoms and signs that may be related to many disease entities. Thus using a decision tree approach based on patient complaints does not provide enough precision to help the clinician establish a diagnosis for patients with oropharyngeal dysphagia.

Gastroesophageal Reflux. Some patients complain of episodes of gastroesophageal reflux (heartburn) associated with their complaint of dysphagia. Some patients describe pain or fullness in the chest associated with their reflux. Others may have reflux and dysphagia but may be unaware that they have reflux because the overt symptoms of chest pain or acid taste are not present.

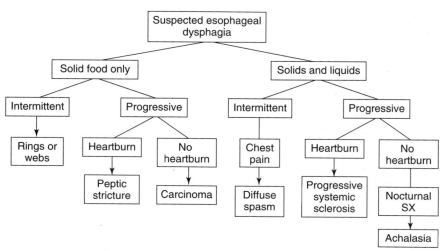

Figure 3-2 Decision tree for preliminary diagnosis of esophageal swallowing disorders. If the patient complains of solid-food dysphagia only, enter the left half of the decision tree and then determine whether it is intermittent or progressive and whether there is heartburn. Follow the similar pathway on the right if the complaint is for solids and liquids.

Not all patients describe episodes of reflux unless questioned by the examiner, because they may not relate their episodes to their dysphagia. This is particularly true when patients complain of globus sensation in the neck, because they might think that reflux in the esophagus could not be related to a problem in the throat (see Chapter 6 for a full discussion of gastroesophageal reflux disease and dysphagia).

Eating Habits. A patient's report of changes in his or her eating habits may signal the presence of dysphagia, its level of severity, and its psychosocial impact. Complaints that center around elimination of specific food items from the diet, such as liquids or solids or items that are sticky or crumbly, may help the examiner focus the evaluation. Excessive chewing of solid food to avoid a sticking sensation may be more consistent with esophageal disease versus the pharyngeal-focused complaint that liquids always seem to come back through the nose. Tiring when eating foods that require mastication may be consistent with neurologic impairment. Patients who report excessive time to finish a meal often have dysphagia that requires careful evaluation. Patients who report that they no longer feel comfortable eating in a restaurant because they have to regurgitate or choke should be examined with care. Patients who have experienced marked weight loss or who no longer enjoy the pleasures of eating probably have dysphagia that has reached a high level of severity.

SIGNS OF DYSPHAGIA

Signs are objective measurements or observations of behaviors that people elicit during a physical examination. In a dysphagic patient who is cooperative, this measurement entails an examination of the cranial nerves relevant to swallowing (see Chapters 2 and 7) and, if appropriate, interpretation of any laboratory findings (see Chapter 8). As noted previously, examples of patient symptoms and corresponding signs are presented in Table 3-1. Some signs are seen during observation of the patient eating. Signs and symptoms may overlap. For example, a patient may complain (*symptom*) of liquid going into the nose and food sticking. Both may be seen by the examiner (*signs*) on the videofluorographic swallowing study. In this circumstance, the patient's symptoms have been confirmed.

The physical evaluation of a patient may reveal signs that are consistent with dysphagia, such as drooling from the lip or tongue weakness; poor dentition; and loss of strength or range of motion in the tongue, jaw, or velum. Poor strength or coordination may result in choking on liquids during test swallows or in lack of bolus flow. The patient's cognitive status may impact swallowing (e.g., failure to chew, talking while swallowing, inattention to the feeding process). Patients who are hospitalized may have more overt medical signs, such as (1) feeding tubes that are already placed, (2) a **tracheostomy tube,** (3) respiratory congestion after eating, (4) requirement of excessive oral and pharyngeal suctioning, (5) eating refusals, (6) undernutrition and muscle wasting, (7) inability to maintain an upright feeding position, (8) an **endotracheal tube,** and (9) regurgitation of food.

TAKE HOME NOTES

- Patients often wait for long periods before they report their dysphagia.
- Patients may not always be able to describe each element of their dysphagic complaint.
- Patients may not always realize that repeated pneumonias and weight loss may be a consequence of dysphagia.
- Symptoms are those aspects of the swallowing process that the patient reports as problematic.
- Signs are those aspects of the swallowing process that are objectively measured and determined to connote a swallowing disorder.
- Not all patients are able to convey their symptoms because of their cognitive status.
- Symptoms and signs of dysphagia may overlap.
- Common dysphagic symptoms include the globus sensation; heartburn; loss of pleasure associated with eating; special preparation, such as excessive chewing; regurgitation; and changes in diet level.
- Common signs of dysphagia include drooling; choking; respiratory congestion after eating; increased need for suctioning; fatigue when eating; poor position when eating; loss of cognitive controls; undernutrition and muscle wasting; and the presence of feeding, tracheostomy, and endotracheal tubes.

CASE EXAMPLE

A 50-year-old woman comes to the clinic reporting a 6-year history of progressive weight loss. She tells the examiner that it has become increasingly hard to swallow both solids and liquids. She denies heartburn. She reports that her dysphagia has interfered with her social life, because it now takes an excessive time to finish her meal. The physical evaluation reveals a right facial weakness with **atrophy** of the left side of the tongue. Her gag reflex is absent and her velum is weak on the left. Her voice is weak and breathy. On test swallows of liquids and solids, she coughs repeatedly.

By the patient's own report, her symptoms of weight loss and a change in social life because of increasing swallowing difficulty seem consistent with a dysphagia diagnosis. On physical evaluation, she has many signs consistent with dysphagia. This is manifest by the involvement of multiple cranial nerves, which has resulted in misdirection of the food bolus into the airway, causing choking episodes that have made it embarrassing to eat in front of others.

CHAPTER TERMS

atrophy Loss of muscle mass
dilation Making a lumen (opening) wider
endotracheal tube A tube placed through the mouth and vocal folds to help a patient breathe
hysteria A complaint or condition that occurs in the absence of any organic disease to explain its presence

motility Movement, as in the peristalsis of the esophagus

obstructive A structural abnormality that creates a blockage, as a tumor in the esophagus might impair bolus flow

organicity Having a medical cause

sensitivity The number of persons identified correctly as having a specific disease

tracheostomy tube A tube placed in the neck below the vocal folds to provide access to the lungs for suctioning and airway patency

SUGGESTED READINGS

Edwards DAW: Discriminative information in the diagnosis of dysphagia, *J R Coll Physicians Lond* 9:257, 1975.

Groher ME: Nature of the problem. In Groher ME, editor: *Dysphagia: diagnosis and management,* Newton, Mass, 1997, Butterworth-Heinemann.

Jones B et al: Pharyngoesophageal interrelationships: observations and working concepts, *Gastrointest Radiol* 10:225, 1985.

Kim CH et al: Discriminant value of esophageal symptoms: a study of the initial clinical findings in 499 patients with dysphagia of various causes, *Mayo Clin Proc* 68:948, 1993.

Lindgren S, Ekberg O: Swallowing complaints and cineradiographic abnormalities of the pharynx, *Dysphagia* 3:97, 1988.

Moser G et al: High incidence of esophageal motor disorders in consecutive patients with globus sensation, *Gastroenterology* 101:1512, 1991.

Nishijima W, Takoda S, Hasegawa M: Occult gastrointestinal tract lesions associated with the globus symptom, *Arch Otolaryngol* 110:246, 1984.

Wallace KL, Middleton S, Cook IJ: Development and validation of a self-report symptom inventory to assess the severity of oral-pharyngeal dysphagia, *Gastroenterology* 118: 678, 2000.

CHAPTER 4

Swallowing Disorders in Patients with Neurologic Disease

FOCUS QUESTIONS

1 Why is it important to possess a basic understanding of the nervous system to clinically manage swallowing disorders resulting from neurologic disease?

2 What are some of the sensorimotor characteristics associated with impairments at different levels of the nervous system?

3 What are some of the dysphagia characteristics that are seen in diseases affecting various levels of the nervous system?

4 What are some of the dysphagia-related problems that are seen in dysphagic patients with neurologic disease?

5 What are some aspects of change in dysphagia over time in neurologic diseases?

6 What are some of the more common treatment issues, decisions, options, and practices in different forms of neurogenic dysphagia?

PRELIMINARY CONSIDERATIONS: SWALLOWING SYMPTOMS AND NEUROLOGIC DEFICITS

Swallowing disorders are symptoms of underlying disease processes. One implication of this perspective is that swallowing disorders in patients with neurologic disorders should manifest the characteristics of damage to different areas of the nervous system. This premise has long been accepted in the arena of motor speech disorders (**dysarthria**). For example, spastic dysarthria results from damage to the **upper motoneuron** system governing speech production. Upper motoneuron damage results in specific patterns of neuromotor impairment: spasticity, slowed movement, exaggerated reflexes, reduced range of movement, and more. The characteristics of spastic dysarthria are believed to be the direct result of spasticity in the corticobulbar system governing speech production. Patients with spastic dysarthria demonstrate slow rates of speech, limited movement of the speech articulators, equalized stress patterns, and other characteristics reflecting the underlying neuromotor characteristics of spastic weakness.

A similar framework helps clinical specialists evaluate and plan treatment for patients with swallowing disorders secondary to neurologic deficit. Patients with damage to upper motoneuron systems demonstrate spastic weakness with resultant slowness and reduced range of movement, which may translate to reduced speed of swallowing (i.e., a delay in initiating one or more components of the swallow) and/or reduced range of movement in the swallowing mechanism (i.e., reduced transport of the bolus contributing to postswallow residue). To understand better the potential clinical applications of such a framework, clinical specialists must be familiar with neuroanatomy, neurologic functions and dysfunctions of various nervous system components, and sensorimotor components of swallowing at different stages of the swallow. Following is a summary of some common neurologic functions associated with various levels within the central nervous system.

BRIEF OVERVIEW OF HUMAN NEUROANATOMY RELATIVE TO SWALLOWING FUNCTIONS

Motor and sensory systems work together to produce movement, including movement associated with swallowing. However, in clinical practice, motor and sensory functions commonly are described separately, because they may relate to impaired swallowing physiology. To facilitate a clinical perspective, a top-down approach to the nervous system follows, in which sensory and motor components are described at each "level." Figure 4-1 is a simplified schematic depicting each level of the nervous system. Table 4-1 summarizes neurobehavioral and sensorimotor functions associated with each level.

Cortical Functions

Functional control of sensorimotor behaviors in the human cortex commonly is described in reference to various areas or regions. The frontal lobe cortex is deemed responsible for multiple aspects of motor control ranging from intent and initiation of movement, to coordination of a movement in time and space, to execution of the movement in an organized and timely fashion. In general, parietal lobe regions are responsible for recognizing and interpreting sensory functions. These functions might include identifying the presence of a sensory stimulus or interpreting a sensory stimulus in reference to an appropriate motor response. Sensorimotor impairments resulting from cortical damage may vary in response depending on location of neurologic deficit, extent of deficit (larger areas of damage are thought to result in more severe or widespread behavioral impairments), and whether the neurologic damage is unilateral or bilateral.

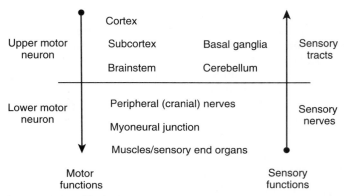

FIGURE 4-1 Simplified schematic of various levels of the nervous system.

Table 4-1	Basic Sensorimotor Functions Associated with Different Levels of the Nervous System	

LEVEL	MOTOR	SENSORY
Cortical	Intent	Recognition
	Initiation	Awareness
	Programming	Motor tuning
	Execution	
Subcortical	Initiation	Motor tuning
(basal ganglia)	Refinement	Awareness
	Inhibition	Sensory conduit
Brainstem	Junction box	Reflexes
	Upper motoneuron/ lower motoneuron	
	Motor/sensory	Sensory conduit
	"Centers"	
	Swallow	
	Respiration	
	Heart	
Cerebellum	Refinement	Refinement
	Inhibition	
Peripheral nerves	Lower motoneuron	Sensory conduit
	Drive movement	
Muscles/sensory receptors	Effect movement	Sensation reception

Other important functions housed within the cortex are human communication and cognition. Damage to primarily the left side of the brain may result in any number of difficulties in the ability to communicate. Focal attention is often afforded to the inferior frontal lobe and superior temporal lobe, although damage to these areas often is accompanied by damage to adjacent motor control areas of the frontal lobe and/or sensory control areas of the parietal lobe. Cognitive deficits associated with cortical dysfunction may present in various forms with different levels of severity and with different clinical courses depending on the location of damage and the nature of the underlying disease process.

The major sensory and motor tracts within the central nervous system arrive at and leave from the cortex. Damage to the sensory tracts arriving in the primary sensory strip of the anterior parietal lobe results in loss of recognition of sensory stimuli in the corresponding body area. Damage to the motor tracts leaving the primary motor strip in the posterior frontal lobe (upper motoneurons) results in paresis or paralysis of the corresponding body area. Regardless of where along the tracts damage occurs, sensory or motor deficits are similar. For example, cortical-level damage to the upper motoneuron system results in the same type of motor weakness as that seen in subcortical or brainstem upper motoneuron damage.

Cortical Functions and Swallowing Impairment

If motor functions of the cortex range from intent to execution, then swallowing deficits resulting from cortical damage may range from no observable swallow activity to poorly coordinated execution of the act of swallowing. In considering these possibilities, common cortical pathologic conditions such as stroke, dementia, and traumatic brain injury (TBI) should be reviewed.

Cortical Areas Involved in Swallowing Function. Before reviewing dysphagia characteristics in various cortical pathologic conditions, it seems worthwhile for the clinician to ask, "Where is swallowing function represented in the human cortex?" Given the complexity of motor control involved in oropharyngeal swallowing, it is logical to implicate the frontal cortex, specifically those areas involved in various components of motor control. In fact, results of both animal and human studies using lesion or cortical stimulation techniques implicate the importance of the lateral frontal cortex, the inferior frontal lobule, and the insula in various motor acts associated with feeding and swallowing.

Although findings from many studies implicate that a dysphagia based in poor motor control results from damage to anterolateral and precentral frontal cortex, no consensus exists concerning the specific characteristics of these dysphagias. However, hemispheric damage to the frontal areas that underpins motor control is a strong clinical indicator of dysphagia characterized by direct movement impairment.

A basic understanding of sensory areas of the hemisphere may be important in understanding swallowing functions and impairments. In fact, studies report that up to 40% of stroke patients with dysphagia may have damage to the parietal lobe. Primary sensory areas of the cortex have extensive interconnections with the motor areas of the cortex. Sensory function is deemed important in the control of voluntary movement. Beyond direct sensory loss, those conditions in which the patient cannot interpret sensory information (e.g., **neglect**) should be considered. Patients with neglect may not respond to a stimulus (food or liquid bolus) in the swallowing tract, not because of direct sensory loss, but because of a cortical deficit in processing and interpreting sensory information. To date, little attention has been afforded to sensory functions in swallowing and swallowing impairment. However, emerging information and clinical observations suggest that impaired sensory functions may have direct influence on swallowing functions.

Issues of Unilateral Versus Bilateral Hemispheric Lesions. Issues previously raised regarding hemispheric contribution to swallowing control also raise the question of whether such control is unilateral or bilateral. A traditional perspective is that patients suffering bilateral lesions demonstrate the most severe and persistent dysphagia characteristics. However, clinical experience and published reports indicate that patients experiencing unilateral hemisphere lesions may demonstrate dysphagia to varying degrees. Recent research using the technique *transcranial magnetic stimulation* has suggested an interesting point of view on the hemispheric representation of swallowing function. Transcranial magnetic stimulation involves sending a magnetic current across the cranium over discrete hemisphere regions. These magnetic currents stimulate motor activity that is measured in various muscles via **electromyography.** This work on the hemispheric control of swallowing function can be summarized as follows: (1) Swallowing motor functions are bilaterally represented in the hemispheres; (2) if the dominant hemisphere is impaired, a contralateral "backup" area may be available to facilitate recovery; (3) a form of **cortical plasticity** may occur over time, increasing the usefulness of the intact, nondominant hemisphere to control swallowing motor functions; and (4) bilateral strokes result in the most tenacious dysphagias. In some respects, this perspective is consistent with traditional clinical observations: Bilateral strokes produce the most severe dysphagias, and many patients with unilateral strokes often recover the ability to swallow after a period of dysphagia.

Swallowing Deficits in Hemispheric Stroke Syndromes. In considering dysphagia secondary to hemispheric strokes, several issues must be addressed. These may be simplified into two general considerations: (1) location of damage and (2) functional consequences of the damage. These considerations are not mutually exclusive. The location of damage may be important in understanding sensory and motor impairments and in understanding severity and potential for recovery based on unilateral versus bilateral lesions. Often, in clinical practice, lesion location information is not available at the time of the dysphagia evaluation. Therefore the clinical examination of functional impairment following stroke provides the best road map to understanding and perhaps predicting dysphagia characteristics. Table 4-1 provides a basic orientation to some of the functional impairments that may be observed clinically following impairment to various levels of the nervous system. At the hemispheric level, intent to swallow may be an important consideration. If the patient indicates such intent, a subsequent consideration would be motor initiation of the swallow. Patients with damage to premotor areas (e.g., supplemental motor cortex) may have generalized difficulty with motor initiation. The clinical picture may be that of a patient who holds a bolus in the mouth for an abnormally long period with associated movements that indicate intent to swallow but without a swallow being initiated.

Patients with sensory deficits may demonstrate a variety of dysphagia characteristics, including retention of a portion of a bolus in the mouth, oropharynx, or hypopharynx with no attempt to clear this residue. Because of the sensory deficit, these patients also may be more susceptible to aspiration of material into the upper airway. Another category of sensory deficit may be seen in the patient with neglect. Such patients may not recognize material presented to one side of the swallowing tract. These patients may be perceived to hold material in the mouth with no intent to swallow, but in fact, they are unaware of the material in the mouth.

Finally, patients with hemispheric stroke may have significant communication deficits or cognitive deficits reducing their ability to relate to the clinical examiner the nature of the dysphagia complaints. Inability to describe swallowing difficulties may delay or hinder clinical evaluation and implementation of rehabilitation strategies. Figure 4-2 offers a graphic depiction of general hemisphere areas that may be associated with various sensorimotor functions associated with swallowing. The left hemisphere is shown for descriptive purposes only. Box 4-1 presents various swallowing characteristics that may be associated with sensorimotor deficits following hemispheric stroke.

A variety of swallowing deficits has been reported following hemispheric stroke. In general, hemispheric lesions (including both cortical and subcortical

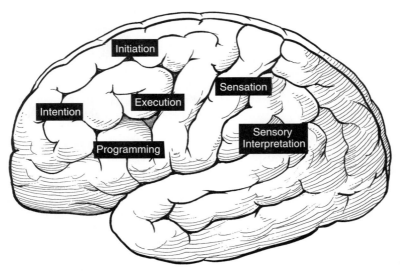

FIGURE 4-2 Graphic depiction of various hemisphere areas that may be associated with sensorimotor functions supporting swallowing function.

damage) contribute to many swallowing deficits, including the following (Box 4-2): (1) poor initiation of saliva swallows (sometimes called the *dry swallow*), (2) delay in initiation of the pharyngeal component of the swallow, (3) incoordination of the oral components of swallowing, (4) increased pharyngeal transit time, (5) reduced pharyngeal contraction and clearing, (6) aspiration, (7) dysfunction of the pharyngoesophageal segment (PES) (cricopharyngeal muscle), and (8) poor relaxation of the lower esophageal sphincter. These collective observations indicate that hemisphere stroke can impair swallowing functions from the mouth to the esophagus. Furthermore, a wide spectrum of swallowing deficits have been noted that range from impaired initiation of the swallow, to poor transport of the bolus, to aspiration into the airway. To date, no report has emerged comparing specific sensorimotor stroke sequelae with specific swallowing impairments. However, the aforementioned list suggests that the array of potential swallowing deficits following stroke is extensive and may relate to the spectrum of poststroke sensorimotor impairments.

Box 4-1	*General Sensorimotor Considerations for Various Swallowing Deficits in Hemisphere Stroke*

- Volitional motor control
  —Initiation difficulties
- Paresis/paralysis
  —Transport difficulties

- Sensory recognition
  —Residue
  —Aspiration
- Communication deficits
  —Inability to describe difficulties

Box 4-2	*Swallowing Deficits Seen in Patients Following Hemisphere Stroke*

- Reduced ability to initiate a saliva swallow
- Delayed triggering of pharyngeal swallow
- Incoordination of oral movements in swallow
- Increased pharyngeal transit time
- Reduced pharyngeal contraction (peristalsis)
- Aspiration
- Pharyngoesophageal segment dysfunction
- Impaired lower esophageal sphincter relaxation

Dysphagia is prevalent in acute stroke, with estimates showing its presence in more than 50% of all patients; however, most acute stroke patients recover functional swallowing ability within the first 1 to 6 months after stroke, whereas a small percentage of patients develop swallowing problems in the postacute period. These observations place high importance on accurate identification and management of swallowing deficits in acute stroke patients. Furthermore, it is important to understand the factors that might predict persistent swallowing problems beyond the acute recovery period. The importance of this perspective is highlighted by the observation that acute and chronic swallowing problems in stroke patients are associated with many complications including dehydration, malnutrition, aspiration, chest infections, and in some cases, death.

Treatment Considerations for Dysphagia in Stroke. Perhaps the most obvious statement about dysphagia in stroke is that it changes over time. From that perspective, dysphagia intervention strategies should also change over time. Table 4-2 presents clinical considerations and decisions that may impact treatment planning over time in stroke. Early in the course of a stroke, focus should be given to basic decisions such as the safety of oral feeding, the presence of **comorbidities** such as malnutrition or dehydration, and the overall medical condition of the patient. As the patient improves and more active rehabilitation is initiated (usually well within the first month after stroke), dysphagia treatment strategies also may change. By this time, a decision about oral or nonoral feeding has already been established and comorbidities are often under medical control. Of importance to active dysphagia rehabilitation are various patient issues and the nature of the swallowing deficit. If the patient is able to participate in active rehabilitation and is motivated, direct and intense swallowing therapy may produce significant benefit. Decisions about which techniques to use depend, in large part, on the specific dysphagia characteristics demonstrated by individual patients (see Chapter 9). Chronic dysphagia is reported in some stroke survivors. Typically, if the swallowing deficit persists beyond 6 months, it is considered chronic. Some reports indicate that certain stroke patients with chronic dysphagia can benefit from intense therapy. Such therapies are typically active and directed at changing specific physiologic features of the swallowing deficit.

Swallowing Deficits in Dementia. Another form of cortical impairment that can impact swallowing ability is the category of progressive diseases known

Table 4-2	Treatment Considerations and Decisions for Dysphagia Following Stroke*
CONSIDERATIONS	**DECISIONS**
ACUTE (0–1 MO)	
Most comorbidities	How to avoid or minimize complications
Resolving dysphagia	Need and readiness for therapy
Malnutrition	How to maintain and improve nutrition
IMPROVING (1–6 MO)	
Patient more stable with better endurance	Need and readiness for therapy
Comorbidities often under medical control	Type of therapy
Feeding routes established for most	
Malnutrition may still be a factor	
CHRONIC (BEYOND 6 MO)	
Feeding routes more established	Therapy or no therapy (prognosis?)
Patients eating orally may have impaired swallow	Type of therapy
Compensations that interfere with swallow	
Impact of prior therapy	

*Changing issues with time post-onset.

as *dementia*. Several types of dementias have been described, with the most common being Alzheimer's disease. Other forms of dementia include multiinfarct dementia, alcoholic dementia, and metabolic and/or nutritional dementias. The hallmark of all dementias is a progressive deterioration in cognitive abilities including memory, judgment, and abstract reasoning, and personality change. Other cortical disturbances such as **apraxia** and **aphasia** might be noted.

Swallowing deficits are well documented in advanced dementia. Persistent weight loss may be the first indication that dementia patients have a significant swallowing problem. Therefore these individuals are at significant risk for nutritional deficits, which may further compromise their health care status.

Characteristics of swallowing function in dementia are listed in Box 4-3. Note that the presence of oral-stage dysfunction is prominent on this list.

Box 4-3	Swallowing Deficits Seen in Patients with Cognitive Decline (Dementia)

- Unexplained weight loss*
- Oral-stage dysfunction*
- Pharyngeal-stage dysfunction
- Combined oral and pharyngeal dysfunction
  —Minor aspiration
  —Major aspiration
- Feeding limitations

*More commonly observed characteristics.

It has been suggested that certain oral aspects of swallowing are under volitional motor control. The generalized cognitive impairments seen in the dementias may contribute to deficits in volitional motor control and hence oral aspects of dysphagia. These may be characterized by lack of initiation of the swallow, in which the patient holds food in the mouth; incoordinated oral control of food and liquid; and/or delayed initiation of the oral component of the swallow, thus prolonging mealtimes.

Although most dysphagia information in dementias has come from advanced stages of the disease, patients with mild-stage dementia also have been shown to demonstrate both feeding and swallowing deficits (Box 4-4). Studies evaluating feeding and swallowing abilities in patients with mild-stage dementia suggest findings similar to, although not as severe as, those reported in more advanced stages of the disease. Specifically, patients with mild-stage dementia demonstrate an overall slowing of the swallowing process from the oral aspects of food manipulation through the response of the pharynx accepting the bolus. This slowing of the swallowing process has direct consequences for increased mealtimes and hence increases the risk of declining nutritional status. In addition, slowing of the pharyngeal response in swallowing may result in reduced airway protection, resulting in an increase of coughing and choking behaviors during mealtime for these individuals.

In addition to overall slowness in the swallowing process, individuals with dementia commonly demonstrate self-feeding difficulties. These difficulties may be noticed in the mild stages of the disease and may become more pronounced as the diseases progresses. In the presence of self-feeding difficulties, caregivers may find the need to offer increased verbal or environmental cues or provide direct assistance to these patients.

Treatment Considerations for Dysphagia in Dementia. Dysphagia treatment options for patients with dementia may range from simple environmental adjustments to the use of nonoral feeding sources. Depending on the specific problem areas in individual patients, possible treatment avenues include the following: special food preparation, diet restriction, taste and flavor enhancement, changes in the mealtime environment, increased mealtime supervision and cueing, or a variety of other behavioral or environmental changes to facilitate increased food and liquid intake. Direct behavioral therapy to change the swallowing mechanics also may be indicated.

Box 4-4	*Examples of Swallowing and Feeding Deviations in Mild-stage Dementia*

Swallowing Deviations
- Slow oral movement
- Slow or delayed pharyngeal response
- Overall slow swallowing duration

Feeding Deviations
- Increased self-feeding cues (specifically related to food preparation or utensil use)
- Direct assistance with utensil use for food preparation or convenience
- Imitation of feeding behavior from the meal partner

Feeding tubes are often recommended for patients with advanced dementias as a mechanism to maintain nutritional support and to avoid dysphagia-related comorbidities. However, the available evidence on the benefit of feeding tubes for this population suggests that feeding tubes do not reduce the risks of aspiration pneumonia, may not prevent further decline in nutritional status, may not prolong survival, and seem to have no impact on overall functional status. More information on using feeding tubes is found in Chapter 11.

Swallowing Deficits in Traumatic Brain Injury. TBI typically results in diffuse neurologic deficits that impact several aspects of behavioral control. Although the incidence of swallowing deficits following brain injury is not well documented, small group studies suggest that up to 60% of patients with TBI may demonstrate some degree of dysphagia in the acute stage. Other reports suggest that recovery of swallowing function in patients with TBI is likely, with most patients regaining some degree of swallowing functions within the first 6 months after injury. Severity of the initial injury may be a strong predictor of both swallowing deficits and duration of recovery.

In addition to the effects of neurotrauma on swallowing ability in patients with TBI, swallowing may be impacted by factors such as the need for **tracheostomy** and/or **ventilator** support, the presence of communicative and cognitive deficits, and the presence of physical deficits that may interfere with self-feeding ability. Tracheostomy tubes indicate some degree of compromise in the respiratory system, which is integral in the swallowing process. In addition, these tubes may have a mechanical impact on swallowing physiology. Patients with communicative or cognitive deficits present additional challenges to clinicians in the design of swallowing assessments or rehabilitation strategies because of the patients' reduced understanding and/or interaction. Finally, physical deficits impose a degree of dependency for activities such as self-feeding and perhaps even for type of food consumed, if facial trauma is involved.

Treatment Considerations for Dysphagia in TBI. In as much as the deficits observed in TBI are multifactorial, the potential treatment strategies and techniques also are multifactorial. Standard intervention approaches include diet modifications, postural adjustments, feeding adaptations, and behavioral maneuvers and compensations. In cases of severe injury with widespread comorbidities, alternate feeding routes may be indicated, especially in the early postinjury course. The good news is that many patients with dysphagia following TBI regain the ability to eat orally with appropriate clinical intervention.

Subcortical Functions

The basal ganglia are a group of cell bodies in the subcortical region that influence the quality of movement. Basal ganglia functions regulate tone (resting tension level of muscles) and steadiness of movement, among other functions. Impairment to basal ganglia functions may create excessive tone and/or extra, unintended movements. Excessive tone may create delays in the initiation of movement, slowed movements, or a reduced amount of movement. Extra, unintended movements disrupt the smooth, coordinated nature of voluntary movement attempts. These may be seen as tremor; regular **clonic movements;** slow, sustained postural interruptions **(dystonias);** or other movements

---

Box 4-5	*General Dysphagia Considerations in Patients with Basal Ganglia Deficits*

- Poor bolus control: involuntary movements
  —Oral
  —Oropharyngeal
- Residue from inefficient swallow
  —Oral
  —Oropharyngeal
  —Pharyngeal
- Difference among swallow types
  —Automatic versus intentional movements
- Severity dependent

---

superimposed on the normal resting state of muscle groups or during intended movements. Box 4-5 lists swallowing problems that may be associated with various characteristics of basal ganglia deficits.

Subcortical Functions and Swallowing Impairment: The Example of Parkinson's Disease

Parkinson's disease (PD) is a slowly progressive disease of the basal ganglia. The key problem is impairment in the execution of voluntary movement. The classic features of PD include **resting tremor, bradykinesia,** and **rigidity.** The cause for this disease is essentially unknown, but the immediate cause for the motor changes is the depletion of the neurochemical dopamine, which results in impaired basal ganglia functioning during voluntary movements. These changes may also result from long-term use of certain medications or may be part of more encompassing degenerative diseases that can influence basal ganglia performance.

Patients with PD may show a variety of interrelated clinical signs. They may demonstrate slowness in cognitive tasks and, in some cases, may display a form of dementia. As the disease progresses, they may show a "masklike" face that appears expressionless. They often demonstrate a characteristic dysarthria, impaired writing (**micrographia**), changes in body posture and gait, and other potential changes associated with reduced movement ability or instability. The progression of PD is variable across patients. No cure currently exists for PD. Medical management primarily consists of medications, although recent efforts of surgical approaches to management have been described.

Swallowing deficits in patients with PD are common and reflect the underlying motor impairments, the extent of the disease progression, and potentially, the effects of medications. In general, swallowing deficits may result from poor bolus control secondary to involuntary movements or from residue or misdirection of the bolus secondary to an inefficient, possibly weakened, swallow. Box 4-6 lists some of the swallowing-related deficits seen in patients with PD.

Swallowing deficits in PD extend beyond the oral and pharyngeal components. Various esophageal abnormalities have been reported, including delayed transport through the esophagus, esophageal stasis, abnormal contractions, and lower esophageal abnormalities. Even further along the digestive tract, patients with PD have been reported to demonstrate **gastroparesis** and various

Box 4-6	*Oropharyngeal Swallowing Deficits Seen in Patients with Basal Ganglia Deficits (Parkinson's Disease)*

Oral Stage
- Lingual tremor
- Repetitive tongue pumping*
- Prolonged ramplike posture
- Piecemeal deglutition
- Velar tremor
- Buccal retention*

Pharyngeal Stage
- Vallecular retention*
- Piriform sinus retention*
- Impaired laryngeal elevation*
- Airway (supraglottic) penetration
- Aspiration
- Pharyngoesophageal segment dysfunction

*More commonly observed characteristics.

defecatory dysfunctions. Again, these irregularities may be related to both the movement disorder and the influence of some of the medications used in treatment of the disease.

It is important to remember that patients with PD must cope with a widespread assortment of daily problems resulting both from the disease and, at times, from the treatments for the disease. These deficits extend beyond the swallowing mechanism and may impact related acts such as preparation of meals and self-feeding activities. In the absence of appropriate support systems, these impairments can have a direct influence on the nutritional and, hence, the health status of individual patients.

Treatment Considerations for Dysphagia in Parkinson's Disease. As with all dysphagias, treatment planning for dysphagia in PD interacts with an understanding of the underlying mechanisms contributing to the dysphagia. In addition, because PD is a progressive disease, intervention strategies are expected to change. Finally, some evidence suggests that medications may have a positive effect on swallowing function in patients with PD. Because medications tend to work in time cycles, it may be important to time meals in relation to the maximal beneficial effect of medications. Table 4-3 summarizes intervention strategies that may be appropriate for patients with PD.

Brainstem Functions

The brainstem is much like a junction box. In the brainstem, the major ascending sensory tracts receive input from the head and neck region via the cranial nerves. In addition, the head and neck musculature receive motor innervation from the upper motoneurons of the corticobulbar system. These upper motoneurons synapse with the motor components of the individual cranial nerves, which function as **lower motoneurons.** Thus damage to the brainstem typically results in sensory deficits to the head and neck region, as well as motor deficits associated with both upper and lower motoneuron damage. Upper motoneuron deficits are characterized by spastic weakness and associated movement impairments, whereas lower motoneuron deficits are characterized by flaccid weakness and associated movement impairments.

Table 4-3	*Summary of Swallowing Interventions in Parkinson's Disease*			
	NORMAL SWALLOW	EARLY SWALLOWING PROBLEMS	MODERATE SWALLOWING DISABILITY	SEVERE SWALLOWING DISABILITY
Presenting features	No observable changes	Reduction in pharyngeal peristalsis Repetitive rocking motion of the tongue	Pharyngeal peristalsis worsens Delay in swallowing reflex Cricopharyngeal dysfunction Laryngeal closure during swallowing may be inadequate	Aspiration both during and after swallow
Intervention	Monitor weight	Provide counseling to bring swallowing under voluntary control	Introduce aids and devices to promote independence	Teach chin-tuck swallowing
	Answer questions	Monitor weight Coordinate eating with drug cycle	Increase sensory input Teach double swallow Recommend small, frequent, highly nutritious meals	Switch to soft diet

From Yorkston KM, Miller RM, Strand EA. *Management of speech and swallowing in degenerative diseases,* Tucson, Ariz, 1995, Communication Skills Builders.

The brainstem also is thought to be home to a "swallowing center" located in the rostral brainstem. This group of nuclei (often focusing on the nucleus tractus solitarius) is believed to facilitate coordination among the various components of the swallowing mechanism (oral, pharyngeal, and esophageal) and to coordinate swallowing functions with respiration. Individuals with damage to this area of the brainstem are expected to demonstrate a severe dysphagia in addition to the basic sensory and motor signs associated with brainstem deficits.

Brainstem Functions and Swallowing Impairment. Swallowing deficits after brainstem stroke provide a good example of the relation between neurologic deficits and dysphagia. In general, dysphagia in brainstem stroke involves two aspects: incoordination presumably related to disruption of the swallowing center and weakness resulting from damage to the corticobulbar system (sensory deficits also may be present). The collective effects of these deficits often are seen clinically as incoordination among "stages" of swallowing and incoordination between swallowing and respiration, as well as weakness in one or more of the muscle groups innervated by the corticobulbar system (e.g., velum, pharynx, larynx, PES). The resulting swallow has been described as the "incomplete swallow." Although *incomplete swallow* is not a specific term, it does offer an overt description of the impairment in swallow physiology seen in these patients. Box 4-7 summarizes features of the incomplete swallow often seen in patients with dysphagia after brainstem stroke.

Treatment Considerations for Dysphagia in Brainstem Stroke. Similar to patients with hemispheric stroke, patients with brainstem stroke recover over time. Likewise, the clinical presentation of dysphagia and comorbidities reveal considerable variability. Given these perspectives, treatment approaches to dysphagia in the patient surviving a brainstem stroke are symptomatic and change over time.

A careful assessment of the components of dysphagia and related deficits is mandatory in patients with brainstem stroke. For example, the patient requiring tracheostomy for respiratory support has a different clinical profile than the patient who does not require tracheostomy. The patient with minimal cranial nerve deficits may offer better physiologic support for rehabilitative efforts than does the patient with multiple cranial nerve deficits. In addition, the nonambulatory patient presents different challenges than does the patient who can walk assisted or unassisted.

In the acute poststroke phase, intervention tends to be more cautious, with a prophylactic component. At this point, the patient may be at greatest risk for pulmonary complications from inappropriate oral intake. Depending on the severity of neurologic impairment and the overall health status of the patient, treatment strategies at this stage may range from nothing (monitoring recovery), to passive sensorimotor activities (e.g., oral hygiene, movement exercises), to more active swallowing efforts involving compensatory maneuvers (e.g., postural adjustments, changes in the swallow behavior).

As recovery facilitates an overall improvement in the patient's health status, dysphagia intervention may be more direct and aggressive. At some point, the

---

| **Box 4-7** | *Pharyngeal Swallowing Deficits Seen in Patients Following Brainstem Stroke* |

- Absent or delayed pharyngeal response
- Reduced hyolaryngeal elevation
- Reduced oropharyngeal contraction
- Reduced pharyngeal contraction
- Reduced laryngeal closure
- Reduced pharyngoesophageal segment opening
- Brief swallow event
- Generalized incoordination (including respiration)

need for continuation of tracheostomy tubes should be addressed. Direct and intensive swallowing rehabilitation has been shown to be effective in facilitating return to oral feeding in chronic patients. The key is for the dysphagia specialist to interact with medical and other rehabilitative specialists to understand the larger health status picture and to select treatment strategies that are consistent with the patient's global needs, while providing the potential for improved swallowing function. $\longrightarrow$ MOT.

The Role of the Cerebellum in Swallowing. The cerebellum is adjacent to the brainstem and is posterior and slightly superior to most brainstem structures. The role of the cerebellum in the control of swallowing is poorly understood. Nevertheless, cerebellar damage results in unsteadiness **(ataxia), intention tremor** (tremor that is exaggerated at the initiation of movement), and **hypotonia** (low muscular tone). When present in the swallowing mechanism, these movement deficits are expected to impair coordinated swallowing functions. Motor unsteadiness and weakness resulting from cerebellar damage may contribute to difficulty in controlling a bolus, difficulty in directing that bolus in a timely fashion, and residue from reduced swallowing effort.

Lower Motoneuron and Muscle Disease

Lower motoneurons proceed through the body and connect with muscles at the **myoneural junction.** Deficits to the peripheral nerves or the myoneural junction produce a flaccid weakness. However, myoneural junction deficits have the distinction that they demonstrate significant deterioration of motor function with use but recover with extended rest.

The endpoints in the sensorimotor chain of events are the muscle and sensory end organs. Motor impairments at the muscle level are called **myopathies,** which are characterized by a severe flaccid weakness within the muscle groups that are affected. Sensory loss may come in many forms, resulting from many neurologic and nonneurologic processes. Reduction or loss of tactile sensation is thought to be particularly important in swallowing problems, because it may lead to unawareness of residual food along the swallowing mechanism or it may contribute directly to aspiration of food and liquid materials into the airway.

Lower Motoneuron Functions and Swallowing Impairment. Amyotrophic lateral sclerosis (ALS) is one disease that reflects the relationship between lower motoneuron impairment and dysphagia. ALS, sometimes referred to as *Lou Gehrig's disease* or *motoneuron disease,* is a progressive degenerative disease of unknown cause. The clinical presentation is progressive weakness, with nearly 25% of patients showing the initial effects of this disease in the corticobulbar musculature. When present, corticobulbar deficits contribute to a significant and progressive dysphagia.

Neurologic deficits in ALS are not confined to the lower motoneurons of the peripheral nervous system. Central nervous system structures also are involved. Therefore the motor deficits in ALS are "mixed," incorporating both flaccid (lower motoneuron) and spastic (upper motoneuron) weakness. The mixture of flaccid and spastic weakness may be seen in the musculature of the swallowing mechanism, in the respiratory musculature, and throughout the remainder of the body. ALS is progressive and terminal, and although many patients survive for longer than 5 years, most do not. Substantial variability in progression rates exists among individuals.

In addition to dysphagia, individuals with ALS experience movement difficulties with the arms and legs, dysarthria, respiratory decline from chest muscle weakness, and in some cases (although rare), cognitive changes (including **emotional lability** and dementia). Obviously, the impact of this disease on all aspects of daily functions is severe. These factors certainly come under consideration in planning any rehabilitative efforts, including swallowing rehabilitation.

Swallowing deficits are progressive and widespread. As might be expected, they reflect a weakness across the muscle groups used to prepare and transport a bolus. General considerations for dysphagia are listed in Box 4-8, and specific dysphagia characteristics are presented in Box 4-9. These deficits reflect limitations in oral bolus control, reduced ability to transport the bolus with resulting residue, and reduced airway protection.

Early in the disease course, no significant dysphagia may be reported. As weakness in the swallowing mechanism progresses, patients may experience difficulty chewing solid food, loss of food or liquid from the lips, and food-specific difficulties. This may cause individuals to begin to reject specific foods or to alter their diet or chewing or swallowing mechanics. As the disease progresses further, patients experience the need for more extensive diet modifications and risk rapid weight loss, indicating nutritional decline. This

---

Box 4-8 *General Dysphagia Considerations in Patients with Amyotrophic Lateral Sclerosis and Associated Sensorimotor Deficits*

- Oral control of bolus
  —Perioral weakness
  —Lingual weakness
- Reduced transport
  —Velar leak
  —Reduced tongue pump
  —Reduced pharyngeal contraction
- Residue
- Airway Protection
  —Bradykinesia
  —Residue

Box 4-9 *Oropharyngeal Swallowing Deficits Seen in Patients with Amyotrophic Lateral Sclerosis*

- Oral stage
  —Leakage
  —Mastication
  —Bolus formation
  —Bolus transport
  —Residual pooling
- Pharyngeal stage
  —Nasopharyngeal regurgitation
  —Valleculae pooling
  —Piriform sinus pooling
  —Airway spillage
  —Ineffective airway clearance
  —Shortness of breath

situation, perhaps combined with the loss of a positive social environment surrounding mealtimes, may lead to the decision to place an alternative feeding source (see Chapter 11). Initially, patients may be able to continue some oral feeding, but at some point, total reliance on alternate feeding sources may be realized. Table 4-4 summarizes a variety of intervention strategies associated with various stages of severity in ALS.

Muscle Diseases and Swallowing Impairment. A variety of pathologic conditions may have a negative influence on muscles related to swallowing function. Typically, these diseases result in weakness in muscle groups that

Table 4-4	*Summary of Swallowing Interventions in ALS*			
	EARLY SWALLOWING PROBLEMS	DIETARY CONSISTENCY CHANGES	UNABLE TO MEET NEEDS ORALLY	SALIVARY PROBLEMS
Presenting Features	Solid foods difficult to eat Longer mealtimes Need for smaller bites	Weight loss Chronic dehydration Loss of enjoyment	Decline in calorie intake Decline in fluid intake Food spillage from mouth Respiratory fatigue	Complaints of too much saliva Complaints of drooling
Intervention	Use chin-tuck position Maintain liquid intake Try drinking through a straw Eliminate caffeine Use double swallow Learn choking first aid Avoid washing foods down with liquids	Change to soft diet Maintain liquid intake Eat calorie dense foods Increase taste, temperature (colder), and texture sensations of liquids	Insert PEG *or* Insert nasogastric tube *or* Insert intermittent orogastric tube	Maintain adequate hydration Use aspirator Use medication Surgically relocate salivary ducts

From Yorkston KM, Miller RM, Strand EA. *Management of speech and swallowing in degenerative diseases*, Tucson, Ariz, 1995, Communication Skill Builders.
PEG, Percutaneous endoscopic gastrostomy.

contribute to dysphagia. The following are examples of disease processes that might impair peripheral muscle function (including the peripheral nerve in some cases): polyneuropathy, myasthenia gravis, polymyositis, scleroderma, systemic lupus erythematosus (SLE), and dystrophy. Each of these is given a brief introduction relative to its potential relationship to dysphagia.

Polyneuropathy. Polyneuropathy, which literally means "pathology to many nerves," may result from many sources. Systemic diseases such as diabetes can result in polyneuropathies as can other processes that impact peripherals nerves. Perhaps most common to dysphagia, and often forgotten, is the peripheral nerve damage that can result from radiotherapy in the treatment of head/neck cancer. Patients treated with radiation therapy not only experience fibrosis in tissue, but also experience nerve deficits in the affected areas (see Chapter 5). Weakness in peripheral nerves innervating the swallowing musculature contributes directly to weakness in the muscles used for chewing and swallowing. Polyneuropathies also may result in sensory deficits with resulting impact on the patient's ability to safely ingest food and liquid.

Mysasthenia Gravis. Myasthenia gravis is a disease process in which the neurotransmitter substance between motor nerves and muscles is depleted with use. In this regard, initial movements (e.g., chewing) often are intact or at least strongest at the beginning of movement (e.g., a meal). With repeated use, the muscles fatigue into a flaccid weakness. Thus any swallowing activity that requires sustained or repeated movement (which is most of them) results in fatigue and reduced function.

Polymyositis, Scleroderma, Systemic Lupus Erythematosus. Polymyositis, scleroderma, and SLE are inflammatory muscle diseases that are more generally classified as connective tissue diseases. Polymyositis (dermatomyositis) is an inflammation of striated muscle. It often is seen initially in proximal muscle groups, and when present in head/neck musculature, it can contribute to oropharyngeal dysphagia. Clinical characteristics may include nasopharyngeal regurgitation, residue in the pharynx, and airway compromise by food or liquid. Deficits of the cervical esophagus also are commonly reported.

Scleroderma (progressive systemic sclerosis) is an inflammation of smooth muscle tissue. In this respect, dysphagia is often esophageal in nature, primarily resulting from dysfunction in the distal third of the esophagus. Many patients with scleroderma experience solid-food dysphagia secondary to esophageal dysfunction at some point in the disease process. However, oropharyngeal dysphagia also may be seen with this disease.

SLE is a disease process that affects women much more often than it affects men. The clinical presentation may vary, because the disease may involve many organ systems. The time course is also variable. Patients may demonstrate proximal muscle weakness (including head and neck musculature), cranial nerve abnormalities, or deficits in the central nervous system. Often, SLE presents as acute deterioration with slow recovery between exacerbations. Many of these patients complain of esophageal-based dysphagias.

Other diseases in the category of connective tissue or systemic rheumatic diseases can contribute to dysphagia. The general presentation is fatigue, malaise, pain, reduced appetite, and often, dysphagia. Dysphagia may present as oropharyngeal, esophageal, or both. Often, the determining factor is which muscle groups are involved.

Muscular Dystrophy. Muscular dystrophy is another category of muscle disease that can affect various muscle groups. One dystrophy that may directly contribute to dysphagia is oculopharyngeal muscular dystrophy (OPMD). OPMD is a slowly progressive disorder characterized by dysphagia, dysarthria, **ptosis**, and face and trunk weakness. Depending on the stage of the disease, dysphagia may be mild or severe.

Treatment Considerations in Lower Motoneuron and Muscle Diseases. Many of the diseases that impact lower motoneurons and peripheral muscle groups are progressive and thus present a special set of challenges to both the patient and the clinician. As with other neurogenic dysphagias, swallowing interventions often are symptomatic, reacting to the specific set of clinical circumstances presented at any given point in time. Various strategies, ranging from behavioral compensations to diet modifications, might be used. The use of strengthening exercises or related strategies may be questionable in some situations. Exercise has the effect of fatiguing muscle groups. If the underlying disease creates weakness in muscles required for swallowing, attempts to overexercise these same muscle groups may serve to exaggerate the underlying weakness rather than to ameliorate it. Thus it is important to understand the impact of the underlying neurologic condition on sensorimotor capability of the individual patient.

Clinicians attempting to improve swallowing function also must remember that these patients are under ongoing medical care. They often are taking multiple medications, and those medications may be changed from time to time. It is important for the dysphagia specialist to have good communication with other members of the health care team who are providing care to individual patients, not only to understand better the impact of various medications, but also to make optimal decisions about changes in the dysphagia management plan. The clinician must also remember that many of these diseases are progressive and that dysphagia management strategies change over time.

Iatrogenic Disorders of Swallowing That Look Like Neurogenic Dysphagia. A variety of contributing factors may create a neurogenic dysphagia in the absence of overt neurologic disease. These factors include undetected vascular deficits (ministrokes), decompensation with advancing age, decompensation in complex medical conditions, medication-induced changes, the initial symptoms of a progressive disease, and postsurgical changes. When dysphagia appears to result from neurologic dysfunction in the absence of overt neurologic disease or damage, the aforementioned contributing factors should be considered. A good rule of thumb is to treat a suspected neurogenic dysphagia as the result of a neurologic process until proven otherwise.

TAKE HOME NOTES

- Dysphagia resulting from neurologic disorders reflects the underlying sensori-motor characteristics of the neurologic deficit.
- Treatment of neurogenic dysphagias is often symptomatic but relies heavily on a strong understanding of the underlying neurologic process. In many cases, behavioral treatment interacts significantly with medical treatment.
- Many neurogenic dysphagias change over time, necessitating different intervention strategies. Change may occur toward either recovery or deterioration of function, depending on the specific neurologic disease or disorder.
- Medical treatments (including surgery) for various neurologic diseases and disorders also contribute to dysphagia.
- In the absence of overt neurologic disease, dysphagia that has a "neurogenic" appearance should be considered to reflect an underlying neurologic cause until proven otherwise.

CASE EXAMPLES

Two case examples have been chosen to represent the more common neurologic disorders that may be encountered by dysphagia specialists.

CASE 1

A 69-year-old man suffered a brainstem stroke 7 months before seeking rehabilitation for dysphagia. The patient takes no food or liquid by mouth; he receives all nutrition by a percutaneous endoscopic gastrostomy. He expectorates saliva into a cup, except at night. Within the past month, he has tasted food but has not attempted to swallow. His anxiety level is high about the possibility of aspiration, but he is highly motivated to initiate oral feeding. He has experienced no chest infections or other complications since discharge from acute rehabilitation. Clinical examination revealed a left facial weakness, but he was able to make a strong lip seal. He demonstrated right body weakness that was greater in the arm than in the leg, and he was able to walk with a quad cane. Endoscopic evaluation revealed slight paresis of the left vocal fold and the left hemipharynx. Fluoroscopic examination of swallowing function revealed incomplete swallow attempts with limited hyolaryngeal excursion, limited opening of the PES (a small amount of material entered the esophagus), postswallow residue for thicker materials, and a small amount of aspiration with thin liquid. He demonstrated a strong reactive cough to the aspiration, as well as the ability to clear residue back into the mouth, where it was expectorated.

Interpretation. This patient is considered to be in the chronic poststroke phase, because it has been more than 6 months since his stroke. He has had no swallowing experience since his stroke, but the observation that he does not expectorate at night (and does not complain of a "soggy" pillow in the morning) possibly suggests that he is swallowing saliva during sleep. The fact that he has tasted food supports his motivation to undertake aggressive therapy. His anxiety about aspiration is understandable and may be a factor to consider once therapy is initiated. The fact that he has had no chest infections and that no history of tracheostomy was reported is an indication of an adequate respiratory system. Being ambulatory is considered a positive sign, because active patients are thought to be less suscepti-ble to respiratory infections than bedridden patients. The alternating hemiplegia (left face, pharynx, and vocal fold versus right body) is characteristic of brainstem stroke. The incomplete swallow is characterized by incoordination and limited excursion of movement of the hyolaryngeal complex, along with reduced PES opening. Material entering the esophagus is a positive finding, as is the strong reactive cough and the ability to clear residue.

This patient is a good candidate for direct, intensive swallowing therapy. An appropriate therapy program for this patient should address airway protection (either by choice of material to be swallowed or compensatory maneuver), hyola-ryngeal excursion (increase upward and forward movement), and swallow coordi-nation (in some cases, slowing the speed of the swallow with prolonged maneuvers may accomplish this outcome). Successful therapy will result in increased oral intake of food and liquid.

CASE 2

A 72-year-old woman came to the clinic with a diagnosis of primary progressive aphasia. The primary complaint was that this woman was losing weight and not finishing her meals. She lived independently and attended an adult day care facil-ity, where she reportedly was observed to cough during lunch. Her brother has a history of esophageal disease, and this was a concern expressed by the family. The patient is ambulatory and shows no overt physical impairments. Her expressive communication is limited to head nods and a few vocalizations but no meaningful words are produced. She is able to respond appropriately to many basic com-mands and requests and is able to participate interactively with a dysphagia exam-ination. Oral mechanism examination was unremarkable, with no overt signs of corticobulbar deficit. Videofluorographic examination of swallowing was com-pleted. The only mild abnormality was the observation that the patient tilted her head upward as she initiated a swallow and that oral initiation and transit were pro-longed. Subsequently, a feeding examination was completed in which the patient was provided a tray of food and liquid (regular grade diet) and was requested to eat. She surveyed the tray of food and promptly began to eat, using her fingers. She was handed a fork and used it appropriately until she faced a situation in which she had to cut her food. She was handed a knife and proceeded to use it as a fork. Despite multiple cues, she persisted to use the knife as a fork and could not be per-suaded to use two tools (knife and fork) simultaneously.

Interpretation. This patient displays features commonly associated with dementias (weight loss, reduced food intake, poor communicative interaction), along with a more rare and specific finding. Primary progressive aphasia is a form of dementia in which language skills are impaired early in the course of the demen-tia, rendering the initial symptoms to be that of a progressive aphasia. The obser-vations of utensil use by this patient suggest a form of apraxia that seemed specific to mealtime and self-feeding. Because, at her age and in her situation, these social functions were central to her life and her well-being, this form of apraxia had a sig-nificant functional impact on her life. The immediate "therapy" for this individual was environmental. The family was instructed to prepare meals that could be eaten with a single utensil (i.e., fork or spoon). The patient was quite successful with this strategy. In addition, it is important to take into consideration the progressive, deteriorating nature of dementia. Although the mealtime adjustment of a single utensil was effective in the short term, as this disease progresses, this patient will require additional strategies to ensure adequate nutrition and hydration. In this respect, her "treatment" plan must contain periodic and regular monitoring of the success of any adaptation used to maintain oral food and liquid intake and the nutritional consequences of that intake.

CHAPTER TERMS

aphasia a multimodal (i.e., speak, write, understand) deficit in language abilities secondary to brain damage

apraxia a deficit in the execution of learned, voluntary movements secondary to brain damage

ataxia loss of coordination of movements, especially voluntary movements; often resulting from damage to the cerebellar system

bradykinesia slow movement

clonic movements spasmodic alterations in antagonistic muscles, which cause a structure to move rhythmically back and forth

comorbidities diseases or clinical problems that coexist with the primary clinical problem

cortical plasticity ability of the cortex to change or reorganize so that functions may be recovered

dysarthria technically meaning "inability to utter," this term commonly refers to one of a group of motor speech disorders resulting from neurologic disease or disorder

dystonias a group of movement disorders characterized by prolonged muscle contractions causing twisting and turning movements or abnormal postures

electromyography technique to measure the electrical activity produced by muscles during contraction

emotional lability sudden and inappropriate change in emotions sometimes seen in patients with neurologic damage; emotional change is out of character for the person and inappropriate for the situation (e.g., crying after hearing a funny joke)

gastroparesis weakness of the gut contributing to poor motility of the digestive system, often seen as poor emptying of the stomach

hypotonia reduced or low muscle tone contributing to weakness

intention tremor tremor (i.e., phasic movement of a body part) that is seen at the initiation of a movement but not at rest

lower motoneurons peripheral motor nerves that course from the cell body in the brainstem or spinal cord and proceed to muscles; damage to lower motoneurons causes flaccid paralysis

micrographia a writing deficit often seen in patients with Parkinson's disease, characterized by very small letters that may be run together

myoneural junction the connection (synapse) between the lower motoneuron (neural) and the muscle (myo)

myopathies pathologic diseases of striated muscles

neglect impairment in sensory processing in which an individual does not attend to one side of the body

ptosis drooping of an organ, most commonly referring to a drooping eyelid

resting tremor tremor (i.e., phasic movement of a body part) that is seen at rest; during movement, the tremor may diminish or exacerbate depending on the underlying neurologic cause

rigidity inability to bend or move, often the result of excessive muscle tone as in Parkinson's disease

tracheostomy technically, the surgical procedure in which the trachea is exposed and opened to create an airway opening in the anterior neck (tracheostoma); commonly associated with a tube (tracheostomy tube) inserted into the open trachea

upper motoneurons motor nerves arising in the motor areas of the cortex and coursing to the brainstem or the spinal cord, where they synapse with lower motoneurons; damage to upper motoneurons contributes to spastic weakness

ventilator mechanical device used for artificial ventilation (breathing) of the lungs

SUGGESTED READINGS

Bath PMW, Bath FJ, Smithard DG: *Interventions for dysphagia in acute stroke* (Cochrane review). In: The Cochrane Library, Issue 4, 1999.

Buchholz DW: Dysphagia associated with neurological disorders, *Acta Otorhinolaryngol Belg* 48:143, 1994.

Buchholz DW: Neurogenic dysphagia: what is the cause when the cause is not obvious, *Dysphagia* 9:245, 1994.

Buchholz DW: Oropharyngeal dysphagia due to iatrogenic neurological dysfunction, *Dysphagia* 10:248, 1995.

Cherney LR, Halper AS: Swallowing problems in adults with traumatic brain injury, *Semin Neurol* 16:349, 1996.

Chua SG, Kong KH: Functional outcome in brain stem stroke patients after rehabilitation, *Arch Phys Med Rehabil* 77:194, 1996.

Clarke CE et al: Referral criteria for speech and language therapy assessment of dysphagia caused by idiopathic Parkinson's disease, *Acta Neurol Scand* 97:27, 1998.

Coates C, Bakheit AM: Dysphagia in Parkinson's disease, *Eur Neurol* 38:49, 1997.

Crary MA: A direct intervention program for chronic neurogenic dysphagia secondary to brainstem stroke, *Dysphagia* 10:6, 1995.

Dray TG, Hillel AD, Miller RM: Dysphagia caused by neurologic deficits, *Otolaryngol Clin North Am* 31:507, 1998.

Egbert AM: The dwindles: failure to thrive in older patients, *Nutr Rev* 54:S25, 1996.

Elmstahl S et al: Treatment for dysphagia improves nutritional conditions in stroke patients, *Dysphagia* 14:61, 1999.

Feinberg MJ et al: Deglutition in elderly patients with dementia: findings of videofluorographic evaluation and impact on staging and management, *Radiology* 183:811, 1992.

Finestone HM et al: Malnutrition in stroke patients on the rehabilitation service and at follow up: prevalence and predictors, *Arch Phys Med Rehabil* 76:310, 1995.

Finucane TE, Christmas C, Travis K: Tube feeding in patients with advanced dementia: a review of the evidence, *JAMA* 282:1365, 1999.

Fuh JL et al: Swallowing difficulty in Parkinson's disease, *Clin Neurol Neurosurg* 99:106, 1997.

Gray GE: Nutrition and dementia, *J Am Diet Assoc* 89:1795, 1989.

Hamdy S et al: Organization and reorganization of human swallowing motor cortex: implications for recovery after stroke, *Clin Sci (Lond)* 99:151, 2000.

Horner J et al: Dysphagia following brain-stem stroke, *Arch Neurol* 48:1170, 1991.

Huckabee M, Cannito MP: Outcomes of swallowing rehabilitation in chronic brainstem dysphagia: a retrospective evaluation, *Dysphagia* 14:93, 1999.

Hunter PC et al: Response of parkinsonian swallowing dysfunction to dopaminergic stimulation, *J Neurol Neurosurg Psychiatr* 63:579, 1997.

Johnston BT et al: Comparison of swallowing function in Parkinson's disease and progressive supranuclear palsy, *Mov Disord* 12:322, 1997.

Kim JS et al: Spectrum of lateral medullary syndrome: correlation between clinical findings and magnetic resonance imaging in 33 subjects, *Stroke* 25:1405, 1994.

Leopold NA, Kagel MC: Pharyngo-esophageal dysphagia in Parkinson's disease, *Dysphagia* 12:11, 1997.

Mackay LE, Morgan AS, Bernstein BA: Factors affecting oral feeding with severe traumatic brain injury, *J Head Trauma Rehabil* 14:435, 1999.

Mackay LE, Morgan AS, Bernstein BA: Swallowing disorders in severe brain injury: risk factors affecting return to oral intake, *Arch Phys Med Rehabil* 80:365, 1999.

Mann G, Hankey G, Cameron D: Swallowing function after stroke: prognosis and prognostic factors at 6 months, *Stroke* 30:744, 1999.

Martin RE, Sessle BJ: The role of the cerebral cortex in swallowing, *Dysphagia* 8: 195, 1993.

Miller AJ: *The neuroscientific principles of swallowing and dysphagia,* San Diego, 1999, Singular Publishing Group.

Morgan AS, Mackay LE: Causes and complications associated with swallowing disorders in traumatic brain injury, *J Head Trauma Rehabil* 14:454, 1999.

Nagaya M, Kachi T, Yamada T: Effects of swallowing training on swallowing disorders in Parkinson's disease, *Scand J Rehabil Med* 32:11, 2000.

Nagaya M et al: Videofluorographic study of swallowing in Parkinson's disease, *Dysphagia* 13:95, 1998.

Pfeiffer RF: Gastrointestinal dysfunction in Parkinson's disease, *Clin Neurosci* 5: 136, 1998.

Priefer BA, Robbins J: Eating changes in mild-stage Alzheimer's disease: a pilot study, *Dysphagia* 12:212, 1997.

Schurr MJ et al: Formal swallowing evaluation and therapy after traumatic brain injury improves dysphagia outcomes, *J Trauma* 46:817, 1999.

Smithard DG et al: Complications and outcome after acute stroke: does dysphagia matter? *Stroke* 27:1200, 1996.

Smithard DG et al: The natural history of dysphagia following a stroke, *Dysphagia* 12:188, 1997.

Strand EA, Miller RM, Yorkston KM: Management of oral-pharyngeal dysphagia symptoms in amyotrophic lateral sclerosis, *Dysphagia* 11:129, 1996.

Young EC, Durant-Jones L: Gradual onset of dysphagia: a study of patients with oculopharyngeal muscular dystrophy, *Dysphagia* 12:196, 1997.

Yorkston KM, Miller RM, Strand EA: *Management of speech and swallowing in degenerative diseases,* Tucson, Ariz, 1995, Communication Skill Builders.

CHAPTER 5

Dysphagia and Head/Neck Cancer

FOCUS QUESTIONS

1 What is cancer? How is it diagnosed? Discuss various impacts that cancer can have on a person.

2 What are the primary treatments for cancer in the head/neck region of the body? Describe several "side effects" that may result from these treatments.

3 What factors contribute to dysphagia in patients being treated for head/neck cancer? Describe some of the more salient characteristics of dysphagia that may be seen in patients treated for head/neck cancer.

4 What are some complications that may be related to dysphagia that are present in some patients treated for head/neck cancer?

5 Discuss the *when, what,* and *why* aspects of dysphagia intervention for patients treated for head/neck cancer. Include consideration for anticipated outcomes.

CANCER AS A DISEASE

Cancer is currently the second leading cause of death in the United States. It has been estimated that nearly half of all men and one third of all women will develop some form of cancer. Millions of people are either living with cancer or have had cancer. These facts clearly indicate that prevention, early detection, and treatment of cancer, as well as appropriate rehabilitation for the cancer survivor, are among the primary health concerns faced today.

What is Cancer?

Cancer is the result of cell growth that is out of control. In simple terms, cells become abnormal and grow rapidly, forming extra, unwanted, and potentially destructive tissue. This proliferation of cell growth is called **hyperplasia.** The abnormality that causes cancer cells results from damaged deoxyribonucleic acid (DNA) within cells. This damaged DNA may be inherited or may result from exposure to an environmental cause such as smoking. The primary risk factors for head/neck cancer (with the exception of nasopharyngeal cancer) have been identified as tobacco (including smokeless tobacco), heavy alcohol use, poor oral hygiene, and mechanical irritation. One potential problem caused by these abnormal cancer cells is that they can travel to various places in the body, begin to grow and proliferate, and replace normal body cells. This traveling of cells is referred to as **metastasis.** This process may occur when cancer cells enter the bloodstream or the **lymph** system and travel to a different part of the body.

Cancer usually forms as a tumor, which technically means a swelling or enlargement, although not all cancers form tumors and not all tumors are

69

Box 5-1	*General and Specific Signs Associated with Cancer (Not Specific to Head/Neck Cancer)*

General Cancer Warning Signs	**Specific Cancer Warning Signs**
• Unexplained weight loss • Fever • Fatigue • Pain	• Change in bowel or bladder function • Sores that do not heal • Unusual bleeding or discharge • Thickening or a lump in any part of the body • Indigestion or difficulty swallowing • Recent change in a wart or mole • Nagging cough or hoarseness

cancerous. Some tumors are **benign** rather than **malignant.** Different types of cancers have been identified that grow at different rates, create different problems, and respond to different treatments. One way to conceptualize cancer is as a group of diseases with different symptoms and signs. Symptoms are noticed by a patient and taken as an indication that something is not right in the body. Signs are also indicative of health problems, but are more definitive of disease as observed by a physician or other health care professional. Signs and symptoms of cancer may change as the disease changes over time. The specific signs and symptoms depend on the location of the cancer; the size of the tumor; direct impact on any surrounding organs, blood vessels, or nerves; and any metastasis of the cancer. Both general and specific signs and symptoms may be warning signs of cancer. These are summarized in Box 5-1.

How Does Cancer Impact the Individual?

Depending on the type and location of a cancer, different problems may be encountered. The clinical signs listed in Box 5-1 provide general categories of problems that may be encountered. Pain is perhaps the most feared of cancer-related problems. Pain does not result from all cancers, but when it does occur, it may result from tumor growth or from the treatments used to attack cancer. Another common problem is fatigue. Like pain, fatigue may result either directly from the cancer or as a side effect of cancer treatment. Box 5-2 summarizes some of the salient characteristics that may be associated with cancer-related fatigue.

Box 5-2	*Salient Characteristics of Cancer-Related Fatigue*

• Feeling tired, weary, or exhausted even following sleep
• Lack of energy to do regular daily activities
• Trouble concentrating, thinking clearly, or remembering
• Negative feelings (e.g., irritation, impatience, lack of motivation)
• Lack of interest in day-to-day activities
• Less attention to appearance
• Spending more time lying in bed or sleeping

Box 5-3	*General Consequences of Malnutrition*

- Increased susceptibility to infection
- Reduced immune functions
- Respiratory failure

- Poor wound healing
- Skin breakdown
- Death

Cancers may also contribute to significant weight loss and impaired immune function. These are not mutually exclusive problems, because malnutrition also contributes to impaired immune function. Impaired immune function contributes to increased complications, poor wound healing, and opportunistic infections. Together, poor nutrition and impaired immune function may contribute to a less optimistic outcome for the patient with cancer. It has been estimated that between 30% to 50% of patients with head/neck cancer demonstrate some degree of malnutrition. Up to half of patients with head/neck cancer reveal some degree of weight loss when they are first diagnosed with cancer. Average weight loss has been estimated between 5% and 10% of baseline body weight. Weight loss may result from reduced ingestion or digestion of food and/or from impaired absorption or utilization of nutrients by the body in the presence of adequate food and liquid intake. The latter situation may be complicated by the need for increased caloric intake resulting from increased energy expenditure in some patients with cancer. Thus some patients have a biologic need for a higher caloric intake, but because of poor food and liquid intake, absorption, or utilization, they actually have a significantly reduced caloric reservoir. This can become a vicious cycle leading to **cachexia.** When weight loss occurs, it may be accompanied by **anorexia,** nausea, constipation, and fatigue. Box 5-3 summarizes some of the more general consequences of malnutrition that may be encountered in the patient with head/neck cancer.

As the preceding information implies, cancer presents unpleasant situations. However, early detection and timely treatment of head/neck cancers often is associated with improved outcomes. From that perspective, it is important to facilitate early recognition of the signs and symptoms of cancer and to obtain an appropriate medical diagnosis early in the course of the disease.

Diagnosis of Cancer

As mentioned previously, the initial indications of cancer are often symptoms identified by the patient. These should not be ignored, because early detection and prompt treatment leads to a better outcome. Depending on the type and location of cancer, various diagnostic tests may be used. These tests are used not only to identify the specifics of the cancer, but also to aid in planning the best possible treatment. Patients with head/neck cancer require a careful examination by a multidisciplinary team of health care providers. Such teams may vary, but a common core membership might include the following specialists: head/neck surgeon, radiation oncologist, medical oncologist, dentist, social services professional, and rehabilitation specialists. The intent of the team workup is to characterize the cancer and to develop the best comprehensive treatment approach (including rehabilitation when indicated). This team may use a variety of diagnostic procedures, including radiographs, computed tomography, magnetic resonance imaging, endoscopy (including both laryngoscopy and esophagoscopy), biopsy and **histopathologic** confirmation, and of course, physical examination. The decision of which procedures to use are often established by the team during review of clinical findings and discussion of options for individual patients.

Staging. A common procedure involved in evaluating cancer is *staging*. In simple terms, staging is the process of determining how far the cancer has spread. This process is important in determining the best treatment options, estimating complications or comorbidities, and formulating a prognosis. Although more than one system is available for cancer staging, the TNM system is used most often. "*T*" (tumor) describes the size of the tumor and extension into any neighboring tissues. "*N*" (nodes) describes any spread of the cancer into nearby lymph nodes. "*M*" (metastasis) describes spread of the cancer to other organ systems within the body. Following each letter, a number or additional letter is assigned to provide more detail. In general, lower numbers indicate smaller, more localized cancers. Higher numbers indicate larger, spreading cancers. Therefore a $T_1N_0M_0$ tumor is small, has not invaded neighboring lymph nodes, and has not spread to other body organ systems. Conversely, a $T_4N_2M_1$ tumor is large, has invaded neighboring lymph nodes, and has metastasized to other body organ systems. Box 5-4 depicts TNM definitions for oropharyngeal cancer. Similar definitions are used for hypopharyngeal and laryngeal cancers; one difference is the inclusion of anatomic subsites for these latter areas.

Box 5-4	*TNM Definitions for Oropharyngeal Cancer*

Primary Tumor (T)

T_X Primary tumor cannot be assessed
T_0 No evidence of primary tumor
T_{is} Carcinoma in situ
T_1 Tumor ≤2 cm in greatest dimension
T_2 Tumor >2 cm but ≤4 cm in greatest dimension
T_3 Tumor >4 cm in greatest dimension
T_4 Tumor invades adjacent structures

Regional Lymph Nodes (N)

N_X Regional lymph nodes cannot be assessed
N_0 No regional lymph node metastasis
N_1 Metastasis in a single ipsilateral lymph node, ≤3 cm in greatest dimension
N_2 Metastasis in a single ipsilateral lymph node, >3 cm but ≤6 cm in greatest dimension (N_{2a}); in multiple ipsilateral lymph nodes, none >6 cm in greatest dimension (N_{2b}); or in bilateral or contralateral lymph nodes, none >6 cm in greatest dimension (N_{2c})
N_3 Metastasis in lymph node >6 cm in greatest dimension

Distant Metastasis (M)

M_X Distant metastasis cannot be assessed
M_0 No distant metastasis
M_1 Distant metastasis

Box 5-5	*Staging System for Oropharyngeal Cancer Based on TNM Descriptions*		
Stage 0	T_{is}, N_0, M_0	Stage IVA	T_4, N_0, M_0
Stage I	T_1, N_0, M_0		T_4, N_1, M_0
Stage II	T_2, N_0, M_0		Any T, N_2, M_0
Stage III	T_3, N_0, M_0	Stage IVB	Any T, N_3, M_0
	T_1, N_1, M_0	Stage IVC	Any T, Any N, M_1
	T_2, N_1, M_0		
	T_3, N_1, M_0		

After TNM description, cancers may be grouped together into stage classifications. In general, four stages are used (stages 0 to IV), but stage IV has three subdivisions (A, B, and C). A lower-stage classification indicates a smaller, non-metastasized cancer. A higher-stage classification indicates a more serious, widespread cancer. Box 5-5 depicts the staging system based on TNM descriptions.

TREATMENTS FOR HEAD/NECK CANCERS

Many cancers of the head/neck region can be cured if found early. Choice of treatment and outcome often depend on many factors, including location and stage of the cancer, the patient's age and general health status, the experience of the medical team treating the patient, available facilities, and perhaps other factors. Although curing the patient of cancer is a primary goal, posttreatment function and quality of life are also important considerations in choosing the type of treatment, because each treatment has potential side effects and sequelae. Another aspect to consider is whether the treatment is intended to be **palliative** or curative. Three primary options are often used in the treatment of head/neck cancers: surgery, radiation, and chemotherapy. These may be used in isolation or in various combinations depending on the type of cancer and the goals of treatment.

Surgery

Surgery refers to removal of the cancerous tumor and some of the surrounding healthy tissue, referred to as the *margin*. Surgery is intended to remove as much of the primary tumor as possible and leave no trace of cancer cells in the margin. However, this is not always possible, and often surgery is combined with radiation therapy or chemotherapy. In some cases, more than a single surgery may be required to remove the cancer or to restore the anatomic or functional deficit caused by the primary surgery. For example, if the cancer has spread to the lymph nodes in the neck, the lymph nodes are removed. This is called a *lymph node dissection* or sometimes a *neck dissection*. In other situations, reconstruction may be required. This involves moving tissue from another part of the body to fill a gap created by the cancer **resection**. A variety of procedures has been described to relocate tissue to the head/neck region. Commonly referred to as *flaps*, these are often named for the location from which the tissue is taken. Therefore a pectoralis major flap is constructed from tissue obtained from the pectoralis major muscle. Other flaps include a lateral thigh

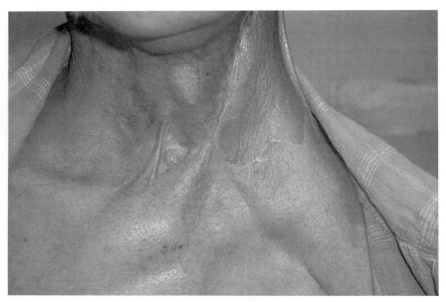

FiGURE 5-1 Photograph of a pectoralis major flap on the left neck.

flap, a radial foreman flap, or similar procedures. Figure 5-1 depicts a pectoralis major flap on the left side. In some situations, bone tissue may be relocated to reconstruct bony deficits in the mandible. If surgical reconstruction is not feasible, a **prosthodontist** may be consulted to construct artificial dental or facial structures to fill a space created by the initial surgery. If the primary tumor surgery creates a risk to breathing, a **tracheostomy** may be performed. If severe swallowing problems are anticipated, a **gastrostomy** may be performed.

Surgery is a primary treatment consideration for all small cancers. Contraindications to surgical removal of a small tumor are the possibility of significant deficits to function (e.g., speaking, chewing, swallowing) or cosmetic defects. Advanced cancers often require a combination of surgery and/or radiation or chemotherapy. Depending on the location and size of the cancerous tumor, various surgical approaches may be used. Box 5-6 lists some of the more common surgeries associated with head/neck cancer treatment.

Surgery, like other cancer treatments, has a number of side effects that can be problematic for patients. Side effects typically depend on the location and type of surgery. Some of these are temporary, whereas others are more permanent. All have an impact on the patient's quality of life. Box 5-7 lists some of the more common side effects from cancer surgery in the head/neck region.

Radiation Therapy

Radiation therapy uses high-energy radiation to kill cancer cells. Death of the cancer cells leads to shrinkage of the tumor. Radiation therapy may be the primary treatment used for small tumors, may be used following surgery to destroy residual small pockets of cancer cells, or may be used before surgery to shrink tumors in the hope of more successful surgical removal with fewer

| Box 5-6 | *Common Surgeries Associated with Head/Neck Cancer Treatment* |

Primary tumor surgery: removal of tumor and surrounding tissue
Mandibulectomy: removal of a piece of the jawbone
Mandibulotomy: splitting the mandible to gain access to a tumor
Maxillectomy: removal of all or part of the hard palate
Mohs' surgery: removal of a tumor in thin slices, with each slice being evaluated under a microscope for cancer cells until all cancer cells are absent
Laser surgery: use of a narrow, intense beam of light to cut out cancer
Laryngectomy: removal of the entire larynx
Partial laryngectomy: removal of part of the larynx: supraglottic, hemilaryngectomy, supracricoid, vocal cord
Laryngopharyngectomy: removal of larynx and pharynx
Tracheostomy: establishment of a hole in the anterior neck (stoma) into the trachea to establish an airway
Gastrostomy: creation of a fistula into the stomach via the abdominal wall, often used to place a feeding tube
Reconstructive surgery: any surgery that attempts to replace missing anatomy to improve function and/or appearance

residual deficits. Radiation may be administered in two ways: external beam and internal radiation. External beam radiation involves aiming a high-energy radiation beam at the tumor and surrounding tissues. A new form of external beam radiation is known as *intensity modulated radiation therapy.* This procedure permits more effective doses of radiation to be delivered to the tumor while hitting less healthy tissue around the tumor. This is intended to result in fewer side effects. Other recent advances in radiotherapy include radiosensitization (using drugs to make cancer cells more sensitive to radiation) and hyperfractionation (giving radiation in small doses several times per day).

Internal radiation therapy involves implanting small pellets or rods containing radioactive material into the cancer or near the cancer site. Patients remain hospitalized while the implants are in place.

Side effects from radiation therapy are common both during and after the treatment. Some of these are transient, whereas others are persistent. In addition, certain side effects may be latent (i.e., they may not appear for a substantial time period [in some cases years] following the completion of radiation therapy). Many of the side effects of radiation therapy to the head/neck region contribute directly to dysphagia. If these occur during treatment, interruptions

| Box 5-7 | *Potential Side Effects of Surgery Used to Treat Head/Neck Cancer* |

- Swelling of the mouth or throat, resulting in difficulty breathing
- Impaired speech and/or voice
- Difficulty chewing and swallowing
- Facial disfigurement
- Numbness in the face, neck, or throat
- Reduced mobility in the neck and shoulder area
- Decreased function of the thyroid gland

Box 5-8	*Potential Side Effects of Radiation Therapy Used to Treat Head/Neck Cancer*

- Redness and skin irritation in area treated
- Permanent change to salivary glands, leading to persistent dry mouth or thickened saliva
- Bone pain
- Nausea and vomiting
- Fatigue
- Mouth sores and/or sore throat
- Dental problems
- Painful swallowing
- Loss of appetite
- Reduced sense of taste
- Earaches resulting from hardening of ear wax
- Hypothyroidism

in therapy may be experienced. Box 5-8 lists several side effects that may be experienced from radiation therapy to the head/neck region.

Before the initiation of radiation therapy, all patients should undergo a complete dental examination. Damaged or decayed teeth may need to be removed, because radiation can cause tooth decay. In addition, patients who receive radiation to the anterior neck region are at risk for damage to the thyroid gland, contributing to **hypothyroidism.** This condition may worsen any feelings of fatigue already experienced by the patient. For these patients, thyroid gland function should be monitored regularly.

Chemotherapy

Chemotherapy refers to the use of drugs to kill cancer cells. These drugs are typically powerful and can cause any number of unpleasant side effects. Chemotherapy may be administered by mouth or intravenously, or it may be injected into a muscle, under the skin, or directly into the tumor. Like radiation therapy, chemotherapy may be used before or after surgery (and/or before or after radiation therapy). In recent years, chemotherapy has been used in combination with radiation therapy in the treatment of certain laryngeal cancers in an attempt to preserve the larynx (i.e., avoid a total laryngectomy) and subsequent voice functions. As mentioned previously, certain drugs may be used in combination with radiation therapy as a form of radiosensitization. Although promising, many combined therapies are still considered experimental. One negative aspect of combined therapies is the risk of more severe or a wider range of side effects. Box 5-9 lists several side effects that may result from chemotherapy in the treatment of head/neck cancer.

DYSPHAGIA IN PATIENTS WITH HEAD/NECK CANCER

Many patients treated for head/neck cancer experience some degree of swallowing difficulty. Some of the dysphagia symptoms result directly from the cancer, whereas others result from the various treatments for the cancer. In

Box 5-9	*Potential Side Effects Resulting from Use of Chemotherapy in the Treatment of Head/Neck Cancer*

- Fatigue
- Nausea and vomiting
- Hair loss
- Dry mouth
- Loss of appetite

- Reduced sense of taste
- Weakened immune system
- Diarrhea and/or constipation
- Open sores in the mouth potentially leading to infection

general, patients receiving radiation therapy (alone or in combination with surgery) are at greater risk for swallowing difficulties than are patients receiving surgical treatments without radiation. Dysphagia that occurs after cancer treatments may be described as resulting from reduced swallowing efficiency. This is characterized by reduced movement of structures within the swallowing mechanism, leading to prolonged duration of various aspects of the swallow and reduced opening of the pharyngoesophageal segment (PES). The reduction of movement during swallowing contributes to postswallow residue along the swallowing mechanism and to poor clearance of saliva. Food and saliva residue may build up over time, increasing the risk of aspiration or necessitating frequent expectoration by the patient.

Dysphagia Secondary to Surgical Intervention

Surgery for head/neck cancer results in the loss, rearrangement, or reconstruction of structures that are important for swallowing function. A traditional rule for predicting dysphagia secondary to surgery for head/neck cancer is the *50% rule*. This rule suggests that removal of less than 50% of a structure will not result in a significant and permanent swallowing problem. However, this rule has been challenged by many clinical investigators, and individual characteristics of patients need careful examination both before and after surgery to identify and manage any resulting swallowing impairment. A general guideline is that the more tissue removed or relocated, the higher the probability for postsurgical dysphagia. Of course, this guideline needs modification in cases in which combined modalities are used (radiation therapy and/or chemotherapy in addition to surgery). Following is a brief overview of certain dysphagia characteristics that may result from surgery to various aspects of the swallowing mechanism.

Surgery for Oral Cancers. In general, the oral cavity involves the anterior tongue, the floor of the mouth, the submental structures, the mandible, and the maxilla. Oral surgeries often involve more than a single structure. For example, a **mandibulotomy** may be required to gain adequate surgical access to tumors in the floor of the mouth or other areas of the oral cavity. Surgeries for oral cancers have the potential to limit mastication, bolus formulation and containment, and bolus transport from the front to the back of the mouth. Surgeries restricted to the tongue often result in transient dysphagia with good functional outcome; however, this may depend on the extent of the tissue removed. When present, swallowing problems secondary to limited tongue resections involve bolus control and transport difficulties.

With more extensive resections involving the tongue and the floor of the mouth with or without flap reconstruction, dysphagia may be expected for varying periods and at various severities. Such dysphagias typically involve problems with mastication, bolus control, transport to the posterior oral cavity, and in some cases, airway protection secondary to loss of control of the bolus within the oral cavity. If the mandible is impaired and reconstructed, mastication may be impaired and loss of oral control is possible. In addition, pain may result from alterations to the temporomandibular joint. In cases of dramatic resection and reconstruction of the mandible, limitations in the PES may result secondary to reduced upward pull from the hyolaryngeal complex that attaches to the mandible.

Surgery for Oropharyngeal Cancers. The oropharynx begins where the oral cavity ends, extending superiorly from the hard palate to the hyoid bone inferiorly. This area includes the tongue base, faucial arches, tonsils and tonsillar fossa, **retromolar trigone**, soft palate, and pharyngeal walls of the superior and lateral pharynx. General aspects of dysphagia resulting from surgery in the oropharynx include nasal regurgitation (sometimes called *nasopharyngeal* reflux), decreased bolus transit, aspiration, and PES dysfunction. Surgery in this area often involves multiple structures, thus increasing the extent of swallowing deficit.

Surgery limited to the tongue base may result in a reduced force applied by the tongue to move the bolus into the pharynx. This can result in postswallow residue in the area of the tongue base and valleculae. Surgery in this region also can result in reduced upward pull on the PES, contributing to reduced opening of this region and postswallow residue in the piriform recesses. In general, surgery limited to the tongue has a favorable outcome regarding the patient's ability to ingest food and liquid by mouth.

Patients who undergo surgery on more than one structure in the oropharynx tend to have more severe and persistent dysphagias. For example, if both the tongue and palate are resected, the patient may experience difficulty propelling a bolus into the pharynx, poor bolus control, and nasal regurgitation. Patients who have extensive reconstruction with flaps may experience swallowing difficulties related both to the ablative surgery and to the flap reconstruction. Flaps used in reconstruction may contribute to swallowing problems because of altered sensation, poor movement, or bulk added to the oropharynx.

Surgery for Hypopharyngeal Cancers. The pharynx is a tubelike structure extending from behind the nose to the entrance of the esophagus. The portion referred to as the *hypopharynx* is that section of the tube beginning at the hyoid bone and extending to below the cricoid cartilage of the larynx. The hypopharynx includes the piriform recesses, postcricoid area, and pharyngeal walls. The larynx rests within the hypopharynx but is not technically part of this structure. The most common site for hypopharyngeal cancer is the piriform recess. The hypopharynx has extensive lymph drainage into the cervical neck region, and metastasis to the cervical neck lymph nodes is common with hypopharyngeal cancer. Thus it is common to see a neck dissection performed in combination with any surgery to the hypopharynx. In addition, hypopharyngeal tumors often do not create overt symptoms early in the course of the disease. For this reason, hypopharyngeal tumors are often advanced, requiring extensive surgery, perhaps involving the larynx as well as the neck. When this situation occurs, a **laryngopharyngectomy** may be completed along with a neck dissection. In some cases, only a partial removal of the larynx is required, and vocal functions may be somewhat preserved. In advanced cancers in this region, reconstruction with a **gastric pull up** or **jejunal transfer** may be used to retain as much swallowing function as possible. Given the location of hypopharyngeal cancers and the common spread of these cancers to adjacent structures (e.g., larynx, neck), dysphagias resulting from surgeries to treat these cancers are severe.

Surgery for Laryngeal Cancers. The larynx may be subdivided into three regions: the supraglottic region, the glottic region, and the subglottic region. Subglottic cancers are rare compared with cancers in the other regions and, when identified, often involve the vocal folds (glottic region). Supraglottic cancers have a higher rate of spread to the lymph system of the neck than do isolated vocal fold tumors and thus may require neck dissection. Both supraglottic and glottic tumors contribute to early overt changes in voice or swallowing and thus may be identified and treated early in the course of the disease. These small tumors may be successfully treated with limited surgeries, including laser surgery. As the size of the tumor and metastasis to adjacent structures increase, the need for more extensive surgical resection is indicated; partial laryngectomy or total laryngectomy may be considered. Partial laryngectomy procedures may include a cordectomy, in which only a true vocal fold (vocal cord) is removed; a hemilaryngectomy, in which one half (right or left) of the larynx is removed; or a supraglottic laryngectomy, in which the structures above the glottis are removed. Figure 5-2 depicts the larynx of a patient after a right cordectomy. Each of the partial laryngectomy procedures may contribute to a reduction in airway protection during swallowing by compromising either the glottic or the supraglottic mechanisms that contribute to airway closure. The extent of the surgery and the functional aspects of any reconstruction (especially in hemilaryngectomy) may be predictive of the presence and severity of any postoperative dysphagia. Patients with total laryngectomy typically are not at risk for airway compromise, because the airway and the swallowing tract are separated. In these patients, a new airway opening is established via a stoma in the anterior neck. Because transnasal airflow has been removed and redirected to the neck stoma, these patients have diminished sense of smell, which may further contribute to reduced food intake. A common dysphagia problem faced by patients with total laryngectomy is **stenosis** in the **neopharynx** created following surgical removal of the larynx. The terms *anatomic stenosis* and *physiologic stenosis* may be applied as simple descriptors of whether this narrowing results from structural (anatomic) or muscle (physiologic) irregularities. Typically, this narrowing of the swallowing mechanism limits the patient's ability to ingest solids foods, although liquids may be swallowed more easily. In cases of severe stenosis, patients may complain of difficulty swallowing both solids and liquids. The videotape that accompanies this text (Crary and Groher: *Video Introduction to Adult Swallowing Disorders,* Butterworth-Heinemann) provides both endoscopic and fluoroscopic depictions of swallowing problems associated with total laryngectomy, as well as a fluoroscopic example of a patient who received a supraglottic laryngectomy.

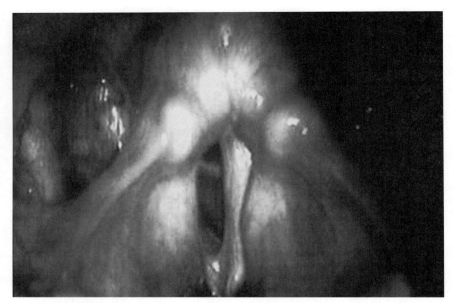

Figure 5-2 Photograph of a larynx following right true vocal cord removal via laser (laser cordectomy). The larynx is shown in the fully adducted (closed) position, as indicated by approximation of the arytenoid cartilages. Note the large glottal opening resulting from the surgical procedure.

Dysphagia Secondary to Radiation Therapy

Radiation therapy in the treatment of head/neck cancer may be used in isolation or in combination with surgery and/or chemotherapy. Radiation therapy may be used as the treatment of choice for small tumors to preserve tissue function (as in the larynx) or for advanced tumors that are not resectable. A general impression is that swallowing problems following radiation therapy either in isolation or in combination with surgery are worse than those seen following surgery in isolation. Radiation therapy contributes to a variety of mucosal and muscle tissue changes, which can complicate any existing swallowing difficulties and create new problems. Box 5-10 lists several complications resulting from radiation therapy to the head/neck region that may contribute to dysphagia.

Box 5-10	*Potential Complications and Side Effects of Radiation Therapy That May Contribute Directly to Dysphagia*

- Mucositis
- Xerostomia
- Sensory changes in taste and smell
- Fibrosis (including trismus)
- Neuropathy
- Changed anatomy (e.g., stricture)
- Odynophagia (painful swallowing)
- Loss of appetite
- Edema
- Infection (fungal, bacterial)
- Dental changes

One or more of these complications occur in nearly every patient who receives radiation therapy for the treatment of head/neck cancer. These changes may occur to both mucosal tissue and to muscle/nerve tissue. Clinical experience with this population suggests that in the early stages of treatment, pain and dryness secondary to mucositis and xerostomia and edema of structures in the swallowing mechanism contribute directly to reduced frequency and efficiency of swallowing ability. Swallowing difficulties that persist or occur following radiation treatment often are linked to fibrosis and/or peripheral nerve deficits. The timing of these tissue changes and resulting dysphagia is variable across patients and is related to many different factors. In general, an intense mucosal tissue response is noted within the first 3 to 4 weeks following the initiation of radiation therapy. Shortly after this point, the patient may be at greatest risk for development of new and severe dysphagia symptoms. If candidiasis (fungal infection) occurs, pain from mucositis may be increased, contributing further to dysphagia complaints. Finally, the impact of radiation therapy on dentition must be considered. Often, especially if the patient has poor dentition, a dentist is consulted for corrective action before the initiation of radiation therapy. Even with this preventive action, the remaining teeth suffer to various degrees from the effects of radiation therapy. Figures 5-3A-C depict various postradiation effects that can occur in the swallowing mechanism.

Dysphagia Characteristics Following Radiation Therapy. General characteristics of dysphagia encountered by patients treated with radiation therapy for head/neck cancer are listed in Box 5-11. The listed percentages are from a single published report and thus should be considered only as estimates. This list contains both contributing factors (dry mouth, pain) and dysphagia characteristics (small amounts, multiple swallows). Only general characteristics are listed. In many cases of dysphagia during or following radiation therapy, pain, dryness, and edema contribute to a reduced frequency of swallowing; misdirection of a bolus leading to aspiration; and/or an inefficient swallow leading to postswallow residue, the need for multiple swallows, and prolonged mealtimes. In addition, many patients complain of a reduced sense of taste, thus limiting eating enjoyment. These factors may contribute to reduced overall intake of food and liquid resulting in threats to what may be an already compromised nutritional state. Poor dentition may further complicate any existing dysphagia by limiting the patient's ability to masticate solid foods.

Box 5-11	*General Characteristics of Dysphagia Associated with Radiation Therapy for Head/Neck Cancer**

- Bolus control deficits (63%)
- Small amounts per bolus and multiple swallow attempts
- Increased meal times
- Reduced frequency of swallowing
- Dry mouth (92%)
- Pain (58%)
- Altered taste (75%)

*Percentages are estimates.

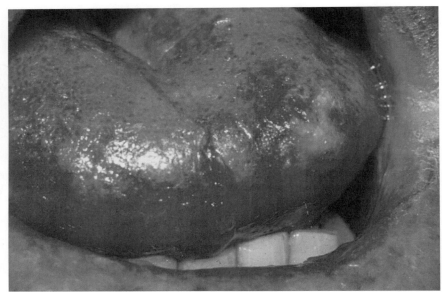

A

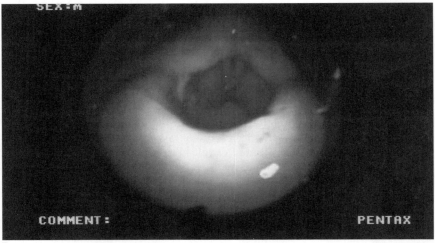

B

Figure 5-3 Postradiation changes to the swallowing mechanism. **(A)** Mucositis of the tongue. **(B)** Edema of the larynx, including epiglottis. **(C)** Persistent and adhering mucus.

THERAPY STRATEGIES FOR DYSPHAGIA IN HEAD/NECK CANCER

Chapters 9 and 10 provide more extensive detail on developing therapy plans and a variety of therapeutic interventions. The patient who has been treated for head/neck cancer often presents a specific set of clinical challenges for

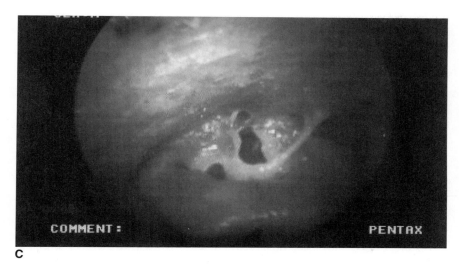

C

FIGURE 5-3 Cont'd.
For legend see opposite page.

therapy resulting from both the cancer and the treatment for the cancer. Most reports of therapy efforts in patients with head/neck cancer are based on small numbers of patients. For these reasons, much remains to be learned about the best therapy for such patients. Many patients, especially those with more advanced cancers, are treated with a combination of surgery and radiation therapy. In this situation, the effects of both treatments must be considered in therapy planning. In an attempt to simplify what may be a complicated clinical issue, bolus transport and airway protection problems following head/neck cancer treatment are the focus of this section. In addition, an overview of interventions that may be indicated to address mucosal and muscle changes resulting from radiation therapy is provided.

Therapy for Bolus Transport Problems

In designing therapy for bolus transport problems, it is first important to identify those changes in the swallowing mechanism that are contributing to the transport problems. These changes may result from either surgical intervention or radiation therapy. The common attribute is reduced movement of the structures composing the swallowing mechanism. Surgical treatment may remove structures that are important to bolus movement. If structures have been removed, a maxillofacial prosthodontist is a valuable resource. In combination with a speech-language pathologist, a maxillofacial prosthodontist can fabricate palatal lifts, obturators, maxillary shaping devices, or other intraoral prostheses that can contribute to improved swallowing function. A palatal lift helps lift the existing soft palate into a raised position, thus creating improved velopharyngeal closure. An obturator is a device that fills a gap created by surgical resection. If the soft palate (or part of the hard palate) is removed, an obturator can be used to facilitate separation of the oral and nasal cavities. A maxillary shaping device is a prosthesis that fits over the hard palate (much like an upper denture). This device may be thickened or shaped to facilitate maximal contact with a weakened or partially resected tongue. Increased lingual-palatal contact facilitates improved oral bolus transport.

In situations in which structures are restricted in movement (from either surgery or radiation), changes in head posture, use of feeding devices, and/or dietary changes may be indicated. Range-of-motion (i.e., stretching) exercises also may be helpful in some instances. Patients who have limited tongue movement may benefit from elevating the chin to allow gravity to transport a bolus to the back of the mouth or even into the pharynx. In these cases, good airway protection is an important part of the clinical picture. If the patient cannot protect the airway and propels a bolus into the pharynx by gravity, the risk of aspiration is increased. Another consideration is that elevating the chin may increase the pressure within the PES. If patients have existing problems opening the PES, this technique may be contraindicated. Logic dictates that use of this postural technique requires a bolus that is amenable to movement by gravity. This may limit the oral diet to liquids or very soft and liquified foods.

Feeding devices have been described that allow patients to place a more solid bolus in the posterior oral cavity. These so-called glossectomy spoons have been used to place soft foods in the posterior mouth in those patients who have lingual paralysis or otherwise restricted lingual movement. In cases of severe movement restriction, patients may use syringes or even soft catheters to place food into the posterior oral cavity, into the pharynx, or in some cases, directly into the upper esophagus. Some patients can learn to pass an orogastric tube themselves.

Stretching exercises may be helpful, especially if approached before scarring or fibrosis is so severe that any movement is severely restricted. Positive results have been shown specifically in increasing mouth opening for those patients experiencing trismus.

Other maneuvers and compensations such as the effortful swallow or Mendelsohn maneuver may also be useful to improve bolus transport in response to specific dysphagia characteristics. Refer to Chapter 10 for a more complete review of various maneuvers and compensations and their impact on swallowing physiology and function.

As mentioned previously, the presence and extent of dysphagia following surgical treatment may depend on the extent of the surgery. This may create the unfortunate situation of "wait and see." Available evidence suggests that effective therapy is early therapy. Research has indicated that swallow function at 3 months posttreatment typifies that at 12 months and that time of initiation of therapy is a significant predictor of therapy outcome. The best strategy may be to initiate swallowing therapy as early as possible postoperatively. Patients receiving radiation therapy may develop dysphagia characteristics during the course of treatment. A percutaneous endoscopic gastrostomy (PEG) tube may be used to maintain nutrition and hydration during and after treatment until oral food and liquid intake can be reestablished. In this situation, it is important to maintain contact with the patient following treatment to either initiate swallowing therapy or reevaluate for oral feeding possibilities.

Therapy for Airway Protection Problems

Airway protection deficits result from compromise of the laryngeal valve. These changes may result from surgical or radiation therapies that impair either the anatomy of the larynx or the movement of laryngeal structures. From this perspective, therapeutic endeavors to protect the airway focus on improved laryngeal closure. In some instances, surgical correction of reduced glottal closure is indicated. Two commonly used techniques are medialization of a nonmoving vocal fold by a technique called *thyroplasty* or injection of a substance (usually fat obtained directly from the patient) into a vocal fold. The determining factors in the selection of the specific technique may be the degree of glottal incompetence, the experience of the surgeon with the respective techniques, and factors regarding the patient's overall medical condition. Figure 5-4 shows the same larynx depicted in Figure 5-2 following medialization via thyroplasty on the right side of the larynx. Note the improved glottal closure.

Various behavioral-therapy techniques have been shown to reduce aspiration during swallowing. These include the chin-down position, the supraglottic swallow, and the super supraglottic swallow. The chin-down position may be helpful when a patient demonstrates a delay in the pharyngeal component of the swallow. This head position allows the oropharyngeal opening to narrow and causes the patient to swallow "uphill" over the tongue. Both supraglottic swallow maneuvers focus on closing the airway before the swallow occurs and coughing lightly to clear any residue in the larynx immediately following the swallow. The difference between these two maneuvers is that the "super" variation includes effort during the breath-hold phase in an attempt to ensure and/or increase the degree of laryngeal closure. The Mendelsohn maneuver may indirectly facilitate improved airway protection by improving swallowing coordination. Head rotation may help protect the airway in some

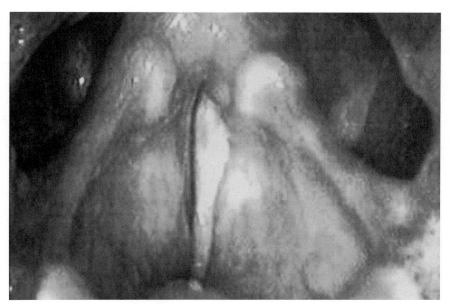

Figure 5-4 Photograph of the same larynx shown in Figure 5-2 following medialization of the right true vocal cord remnant via thyroplasty. Note the improved glottal closure by comparing the two photographs.

patients, especially in those with hemipharyngeal deficits, by redirecting the bolus to the more intact side of the pharynx. Refer to Chapter 10 for more information on these therapy maneuvers.

Therapies for Mucosal and Muscle Changes Resulting from Radiation Treatments

When radiation therapy creates mucosal and muscle tissue changes that interfere with swallowing, it is in the patient's best interest for the therapy plan to incorporate activities directed at minimizing the impact of those tissue changes. Box 5-12 summarizes some of the more common interventions for both mucosal and muscle tissue changes created by radiation therapy in the treatment of head/neck cancer.

Xerostomia, or dry mouth, can contribute to swallowing difficulties as a result of reduced watery saliva that mixes with food to assist in bolus transport. Anyone who has tried to swallow repeatedly without attempts to generate more saliva will recognize the impact that a severely dry mouth has on swallowing function. Another function of saliva is to promote improved oral and dental health; reduced salivary flow can contribute to impaired oral and dental health. Synthetic salivas are commercially available as a replacement for lost natural saliva. These come in various forms, including mouthwash, sprays, gels, and even chewing gum. Experience has shown that some patients use and benefit from these materials, whereas others reject them. Many patients report using a water spritzer bottle that they carry with them to use for dry mouth as needed. These patients also frequently use liquids during meals to help transport food through the swallowing mechanism and to remove postswallow residue. Of course, this strategy requires adequate airway protection to minimize or eliminate risk of aspiration. Physicians may prescribe medication to increase salivary flow. These medications tend to require extended use, and the cost may be prohibitive for some patients. These medications also increase fluid secretion from many glands in addition to that from salivary glands. Some patients report profuse sweating when taking these medications. In reality, many patients experiencing xerostomia experiment with different approaches to improving oral "lubrication." Clinicians can help this process by providing a wide range of options and information. One consideration for the patient with xerostomia is oral hygiene. Reduction of saliva has the potential to compromise oral and dental health. Clinicians should counsel patients to engage in a routine of frequent oral hygiene activities that are consistent with the condition of the oral cavity.

Box 5-12	*Common Interventions for Mucosal and Muscle Changes Resulting from Radiation Therapy for Head/Neck Cancer*

Mucosal Changes
- Salivary supplements
- Water
- Analgesics
- Ice chips
- Mouthwash
- Gels
- Prescription medications
- Mechanical cleansing

Muscle Changes
- Cold (including ice chips)
- Stretching activities
- Various exercises

Oral pain may result from mucositis. In severe cases, this pain can be excruciating and can cause the individual to reduce the frequency of swallowing or cease oral intake of food and liquid altogether. Few proven strategies are available to combat this situation. A recent review of the evidence in this area suggests that the strongest support exists for using ice chips during the course of radiation therapy. Another strategy that has some support is mechanical cleansing with saline (brushing the tongue and oral structures with salt water and a very soft toothbrush). Some patients report using oral analgesic gels similar to those used for babies who are cutting their first teeth. In cases of very severe pain, physicians may prescribe analgesic patches of strong pain-suppressing medication. In milder cases, an over-the-counter liquid medication may be adequate to suppress pain.

Changes in muscle tissue occur in the direction of restricted movement of structures resulting from fibrosis or neuropathy in muscles that have been radiated. No single therapy has been shown to be a panacea for all patients. Consultation with a physical therapist may be valuable to identify strategies to increase movement in fibrotic muscles. One general strategy is to stretch the restricted structure and thereby the fibrotic muscles. Repetitive stretching has been shown to improve movement, especially in the jaw. Both commercial and "home-grown" devices are available to facilitate this approach.

In severe cases of radiation changes in mucosa or muscle tissue, patients cannot maintain any oral intake of food or liquid. In these cases, the physician providing the cancer treatment may opt for nonoral feeding strategies. Available evidence supports the use of a PEG tube over a nasogastric tube. PEG feedings have been shown to be superior to nasogastric feeding in reference to less mechanical failure, better nutritional outcomes, and fewer associated chest infections in this patient population. The decision to pursue nonoral feeding strategies is typically based on individual patient circumstances and is often done in consultation with a dietitian and a speech-language pathologist. As mentioned previously, it is important to follow these patients over time to determine whether oral feeding may be reestablished or whether swallowing therapy may be beneficial.

TAKE HOME NOTES

- Cancer within the swallowing mechanism and the treatments for cancer contribute to dysphagia and other life-altering changes. The primary treatments for cancer are surgery and radiation therapy. These may be used alone or in combination. Chemotherapy may be used in combination with one of these primary approaches.
- Dysphagia characteristics resulting from treatments for head/neck cancer vary depending on the type and extent of the treatment. One common feature is reduced movement within the swallowing mechanism. This contributes to reduced swallowing efficiency, which may be observed in many ways. Knowledge of the nature and extent of the cancer treatment is helpful in understanding and developing therapeutic strategies for resulting dysphagia.
- Patients who receive radiation therapy in isolation or in combination with surgery may experience dysphagia related to reduced movement of structures within the swallowing mechanism and/or secondary to pain and

dryness in the oropharyngeal structures. If dysphagia is present, these treatment complications may require direct intervention to facilitate improved swallowing function.

- In evaluating swallowing function in the patient who has been treated for head/neck cancer, it is important to evaluate dysphagia-related conditions including nutritional status, senses of taste and smell, endurance, and oral pain.
- Therapy for dysphagia in patients with head/neck cancer often focuses on bolus transport issues and airway protection issues. A variety of surgical and behavioral therapy strategies is available to improve swallowing function. Recent research has suggested that the earlier therapy is initiated, the better the expected outcome.

CASE EXAMPLE

The patient is a 66-year-old man status post left neck dissection and radiation therapy for cancer of the left tonsillar fossa ($T_2N_{2a}M_0$). He completed radiation therapy 4 months before his first visit to the outpatient dysphagia clinic. A left neck dissection was planned following radiation therapy; however, at the completion of radiation therapy the patient acquired pneumonia, which was presumed to be related to aspiration, and was hospitalized for treatment. A PEG tube was placed during that hospital stay. During that hospitalization, a fluorographic swallowing evaluation revealed no aspiration. A left neck dissection was completed 2 months later (2 months before presentation to dysphagia clinic). A repeat fluorographic study showed aspiration 3 weeks following this surgery, and it was recommended that the patient take only thickened liquids. He came to the outpatient dysphagia clinic 4 weeks later. Endoscopic assessment of swallowing functions identified no aspiration of thin liquids. Penetration of thick liquids was noted and they were effectively cleared with a cough. He showed moderate post–radiation therapy changes in the pharynx, including reduced movement of the pharyngeal wall during falsetto, adhering mucus in the pharynx, and postswallow residue that increased as the viscosity of the bolus increased. A subsequent fluorographic study indicated better swallowing performance (no aspiration, less residue) with thin liquids than with thicker materials. Swallow movements were deemed adequate to support functional swallowing but reduced in degree of movement (reduced hyolaryngeal elevation, reduced pharyngeal contraction, and reduced PES opening). The recommendation at that time was to initiate oral intake of thin liquids and to gradually increase viscosity as tolerated up to a soft food consistency. He was to be followed by his local physician and a speech-language pathologist.

This patient was again hospitalized 10 months later with right lower lobe pneumonia. At that time, fluorographic study indicated aspiration, and it was recommended that the patient cease all oral intake of food or liquid. He again presented to the dysphagia clinic 2 months later. Fluorographic study indicated aspiration when the patient attempted to swallow 10 ml of thick liquid, but not when he attempted to swallow thin liquid or smaller volumes of thick liquid (5 ml). Both a supraglottic swallow and a Mendelsohn maneuver were taught, and both were successful in reducing or eliminating aspiration during larger-bolus swallows. At this point, intensive swallowing therapy was recommended with a focus on airway protection and increasing hyolaryngeal elevation, pharyngeal contraction, and PES opening during swallowing. The Mendelsohn maneuver with increasing effort was emphasized, and a progression of materials beginning with thin liquid, progressing to thick liquids and pureed foods, was introduced. Surface electromyography biofeedback was used to teach the maneuver and to monitor increased swallowing effort. Postswallow airway clearance was monitored with cervical auscultation.

After 2 weeks of daily therapy sessions, the patient demonstrated increased base of tongue contact to the posterior pharyngeal wall, increased extent and duration of pharyngeal contraction, and increased hyolaryngeal elevation. He was able to take in larger volumes of thin liquid without aspiration (cup drinking) and demonstrated less residue with swallows of thick liquid. After 2 additional weeks of daily therapy, this patient was able to ingest thickened liquids without aspiration and with minimal residue, and he was able to ingest "moist puree" foods with only minimal residue and no signs of aspiration. At this point, he met with the team dietitian to discuss strategies for increasing intake to total oral feeding while reducing tube feedings. Subsequently, his PEG tube was removed and he returned to total oral intake of food and liquid. His diet was restricted to liquids and soft foods, but he reported that this was indeed better for him than tube feedings.

Points to Consider This patient represents a case of moderate reduction of movement within the swallowing mechanism secondary to radiation therapy. His case was somewhat complicated by the appearance of pneumonia following completion of radiation therapy and by the inconsistent findings of aspiration across instrumental examinations. This inconsistency might result from variability within the patient over time or from variability in how these examinations were completed (see Chapter 8). One consistent finding was that he swallowed thin liquid better than thicker materials. This may result from less force applied to a bolus secondary to reduced movement of structures within the swallowing tract or perhaps secondary to xerostomia, which creates more adherence between oral mucosa and thicker materials. The initial approach to increase oral intake for this patient was to start him on material deemed safe based on instrumental study and allow him to progress at his own pace under supervision of his physician and local therapist. This was somewhat successful, but the level of intensity of his attempts and his compliance with a routine were unknown with this approach. The subsequent therapy program for this patient focused on attempting to increase movement of oropharyngeal structures during swallowing attempts while taking precaution to reduce the risk of aspiration of material into the airway. In this case, he improved, although it was more than 1 year following radiation therapy. Possibly because he was continuing to swallow during this period, some flexibility in the mechanism was retained or at least not compromised further. This case presents many interesting questions, not all of which can be answered directly. However, this case does demonstrate that swallowing rehabilitation can be successful and safe even in patients who present chronic conditions and who are at risk for airway compromise.

CHAPTER TERMS

anorexia loss of appetite
benign not recurrent or progressive; nonmalignant
cachexia a state of ill health, malnutrition, and wasting

gastric pull up a surgical technique in which the stomach is raised into the thorax, often with reconnection to the swallowing mechanism in the hypopharynx

gastrostomy the creation of a fistula through the abdominal wall; often used in reference to feeding tubes placed through a fistula placed through the abdominal wall into the stomach

histopathologic the microscopic evaluation of diseased tissues

hyperplasia excessive proliferation of cells

hypothyroidism a condition caused by deficient thyroid secretion resulting in lowered basal metabolism

jejunal transfer replacing part of the esophagus and/or hypopharynx with a portion of the jejunum (a portion of the small intestine)

laryngopharyngectomy removal of the larynx and pharynx

lymph a fluid system containing vessels and nodes throughout the body; lymph fluid is formed all over the body but eventually enters the thoracic area where it enters the bloodstream

malignant growing worse or resisting treatment; tending or threatening to produce death

mandibulotomy procedure in which a portion of the mandible is split or opened to gain access to other structures and is then closed

metastasis movement of cells from one part of the body to another

neopharynx "new pharynx"; a term referring to the reorganized pharynx following total laryngectomy

palliative relieving symptoms without curing the disease; sometimes refers to reducing discomfort in patients with terminal disease

prosthodontist a dentist trained in making artificial teeth and other maxillo-facial structures

resection "cutting off"; partial removal of a structure

retromolar trigone area behind the molars

stenosis narrowing

tracheostomy procedure in which an opening (stoma) is made in the anterior neck into the trachea to establish an airway

SUGGESTED READINGS

Body JJ: The syndrome of anorexia-cachexia, *Curr Opin Oncol* 11:255, 1999.

Colangelo L, Logemann J, Rademaker A: Tumor size and pretreatment speech and swallowing in patients with respectable tumors, *Otolaryngol Head Neck Surg* 122: 653, 2000.

Collins MM, Wight RG, Partridge G: Nutritional consequences of radiotherapy in early laryngeal carcinoma, *Ann R Coll Surg Engl* 81:376, 1999.

Denk DM et al: Prognostic factors for swallowing rehabilitation following head and neck cancer surgery, *Acta Otolaryngol* 117:769, 1997.

Denk DM, Kaider A: Videoendoscopic biofeedback: a simple method to improve the efficacy of swallowing rehabilitation of patients after head and neck surgery, *Otorhinolaryngol* 59:100, 1997.

Epstein JB et al: Quality of life and oral function following radiotherapy for head and neck cancer, *Head Neck* 21:1, 1999.

Fietkau R: Principles of feeding cancer patients via enteral or parenteral nutrition during radiotherapy, *Strahlenther Onkol* 174(Suppl):47, 1998.

Fleming SM: Treatment for mechanical swallowing disorders. In Groher ME, ed: *Dysphagia diagnosis and management,* ed 3, Boston, 1997, Butterworth-Heineman

Groher ME: Mechanical disorders of swallowing. In Groher ME, editor: *Dysphagia diagnosis and management,* ed 3, Boston, 1997, Butterworth-Heinemann.

Kendall K et al: Timing of swallowing events after single-modality treatment of head and neck carcinomas with radiotherapy, *Head Neck* 20:720, 1998.

Lee JH et al: Prophylactic gastrostomy tubes in patients undergoing intensive irradiation for cancer of the head and neck, *Arch Otolaryngol Head Neck Surg* 124:871, 1998.

Logemann J et al: Supersupraglottic swallow in irradiated head and neck cancer patients, *Head Neck* 19:535, 1997.

Magne N et al: Comparison between nasogastric tube feeding and percutaneous fluoroscopic gastrostomy in advanced head and neck cancer patients, *Eur Arch Otorhinolaryngol* 258:89, 2001.

Medina JE, Khafif A: Early oral feeding following total laryngectomy, *Laryngoscope* 111:368, 2001.

Mekhail TM et al: Enteral nutrition during the treatment of head and neck carcinoma: is a percutaneous endoscopic gastrostomy tube preferable to a nasogastric tube? *Cancer* 91:1785, 2001.

Meuric J et al: Good clinical practice in nutritional management of head and neck cancer patients, *Bull Cancer* 86:843, 1999.

Pauloski B, Logemann J, Rademker A: Speech and swallowing function after oral and oropharyngeal resections: one year follow up, *Head Neck* 16: 313, 1994.

Pauloski B et al: Pretreatment swallowing function in patients with head and neck cancer, *Head Neck* 22:474, 2000.

Symonds RP: Treatment-induced mucositis: an old problem with new remedies, *Br J Cancer* 77:1689, 1998.

van Bokhorst-de van der Schuer et al: The impact of nutritional status on the prognoses of patients with advanced head and neck cancer, *Cancer* 86:519, 1999.

Zuydam A et al: Swallowing rehabilitation after oro-pharyngeal resection for squamous cell carcinoma, *Br J Oral Maxillo Surg* 38:513, 2000.

CHAPTER 6

Esophagopharyngeal Disorders

FOCUS QUESTIONS

1   Why is it important to recognize that primary esophageal swallowing disorders may affect oropharyngeal function?
2   What are some potential disorders of swallowing that affect the esophagus that also may affect pharyngeal swallowing function?
3   What is gastroesophageal reflux disease (GERD)?
4   What are the potential effects of GERD on the esophagus, pharynx, larynx, and mouth?

ESOPHAGOPHARYNGEAL DISORDERS

It is important to recognize interrelationships of function between the esophagus, pharynx, and mouth. Without this understanding, treatable disorders of swallowing may go undetected. Primary disorders in one stage of swallowing may have secondary effects on another stage. For example, gastroesophageal reflux that reaches the level of the pharynx may affect the mechanics of the pharyngoesophageal segment (PES), or a disorder that results in bolus stasis in the pharynx might interfere with esophageal peristalsis, because the strength of primary esophageal peristalsis depends on the complete emptying of the esophagus (see Chapter 2). Although a primary disorder in one stage of swallow may affect another stage, a cause and effect relationship rarely is experimentally established. Nonetheless, patients who complain of food sticking at the level of the neck and who have a normal swallowing study of that region should have laboratory studies to rule out esophageal pathology as the primary site of the disorder. The speech-language pathologist often receives referrals on patients with suspected pharyngeal swallowing impairment who have an esophageal disorder as the primary cause. Management of these patients is facilitated if the clinician maintains a perspective that, functionally, the aerodigestive tract is one unit.

GASTROESOPHAGEAL REFLUX DISEASE

Gastroesophageal reflux disease (GERD), commonly referred to as *heartburn*, affects between 30% and 50% of the U.S. population. However, not all patients with GERD complain of heartburn, and not all patients with heartburn complain of dysphagia. Nevertheless, GERD may be the source of dysphagia that has the potential to affect all stages of swallowing. Theoretically, GERD can affect swallowing by two mechanisms: (1) by direct contact of acid on the mucosa that lines the aerodigestive tract and (2) by acidic irritation of cranial nerve (CN) X, which innervates most of the aerodigestive tract.

What Is GERD?

GERD is the free flow of acidic (hydrochloric) gastric contents into the esophagus through the lower esophageal sphincter (LES). GERD is a common physiologic occurrence and in most persons does not cause symptoms or signs of tissue damage. However, it can cause damage to the aerodigestive tract mucosa. When GERD is severe, acid can reach the level of the PES, enter the pharynx and/or larynx, or reach the mouth. When this acid is aspirated into the lungs, a chemical **pneumonitis** may result. Gastric contents may flow back into these areas for a variety of reasons. These reasons include (1) failure of the LES to maintain sufficient closure pressures; (2) high, positive intragastric pressures that allow fluid to flow into the negative esophageal pressure zone; (3) the presence of a nasogastric tube that artificially opens the sphincter; and (4) transient lower esophageal sphincter relaxations (tLESRs). It is thought that tLESRs, which are present in all persons, are the genesis for most events of reflux. These events often are not associated with eating, but rather with pressure alterations in the LES during changes in respiratory demand or in changes of position, such as bending or lifting. The secondary effects of GERD may result in dysphagia that causes the patient to seek medical attention. In some cases, dysphagia is the presenting symptom and GERD is identified as the primary cause.

GERD and the Esophagus

Acid that is refluxed into the esophagus may result in numerous esophageal pathologic conditions, some of which may have secondary effects on oropharyngeal function. These conditions include (1) esophagitis, (2) esophagitis with stricture, and (3) precancerous mucosal changes **(Barrett's esophagus).**

Esophagitis. When acid frequently comes into contact with the mucosal lining of the esophagus, the potential for the mucosa to become inflamed is high. Evidence suggests that this irritation may result in loss of esophageal motility, either from vagal (CN X) irritation or from secondary **edema** that interferes with the peristalsis of the esophagus. It is conceivable that patients with poor esophageal motility may complain of food sticking at the level of the neck.

Esophagitis with Stricture. Severe esophagitis may result in the formation of a stricture that obstructs the flow of food. The esophagus often becomes distended and immobile above the level of the stricture. The distension impairs peristalsis and therefore impairs normal motility. Patients often claim that food is sticking in their chest; however, those symptoms also may be felt in the neck. Severe strictures may result in the regurgitation of food or fluid.

Barrett's Esophagus. Barrett's esophagus results from an inflammation of the cells in the region of the LES. GERD and chemotherapy are potential sources for this irritation. Cellular **dysplasia** in the LES may result in a cancerous tumor that produces obstruction with dysmotility and dysphagia. Removal of the esophagus (i.e., esophagectomy) secondary to cancer often affects the mechanics of the entire aerodigestive tract.

GERD and the PES

Acid that reaches the level of the PES may interfere with the normal physiology of this region, although this notion awaits experimental verification. It is conceivable that the irritative effects of acid have the potential to precipitate **muscle hypertrophy, fibrosis,** degeneration, or other tissue changes. These changes may result in dysphagia from either obstruction or failure in PES relaxation or closure. Because the entrance to the airway is in close proximity to this region, food or fluid that is retained above the PES or that is refluxed through the PES from below may cause tracheal aspiration.

Cricopharyngeal Bar. The cricopharyngeal muscle is located in the middle of the PES at the level of the cervical esophagus (see Figure 2-4). The presence of this muscle as viewed during videofluorographic swallowing studies may be more prominent in those who complain of dysphagia. However, it can be seen as a normal variation in people who are not dysphagic. This patient had no complaints of dysphagia. An example of a more prominent cricopharyngeal sphincter that results in a narrowing of the opening into the esophagus is shown in Figure 6-1. In this position, the muscle has the appearance of a "bar" or ledge. This example of cricopharyngeal muscle hypertrophy caused the patient to have swallowing complaints. There is no evidence to suggest that the length of the bar (percentage of cricopharyngeal muscle indentation) correlates with dysphagia severity. The cause of the cricopharyngeal bar remains speculative and includes esophageal-related disorders with or without GERD and neurogenic disorders, such as stroke, that affect striated muscle. Some investigators have noted that the cricopharyngeal bar produces dysphagic symptoms only if the cricopharyngeal hypertrophy is seen throughout the entire swallowing sequence during videofluorography.

Some investigators have not attributed the cricopharyngeal bar to a hypertrophy of the muscle but to a failure of the muscle to relax and contract. In effect, bolus flow is blocked temporarily because of cricopharyngeal "spasm." Use of the term *spasm* is controversial when a prominent cricopharyngeal sphincter that inhibits bolus flow is seen, because it may not represent true muscle spasm. Because the stenosis is one of physiologic abnormality, it may be best characterized as a **physiologic stenosis.** Physiologic stenosis describes the temporary resistance to flow seen in disorders of the PES that are initially obstructive but that yield to bolus flow. An example of physiologic stenosis can be seen in the videotape that accompanies this text (Crary and Groher, *Video Introduction to Adult Swallowing Disorders,* Butterworth-Heinemann).

PES Fibrosis. Fibrosis is a change in the connective tissue of muscle that results in a stiffening or lack of mobility of that muscle. When fibrosis is severe, the muscle is rendered immobile. It is conceivable that the secondary inflammatory effects of GERD to the level of the PES can precipitate muscle fibrosis. More commonly, the side effects from radiation treatments may result in muscle fibrosis. Another cause of fibrosis is scarring from surgery. Fibrotic changes in the PES may result in a stenosis similar to the one seen in cricopharyngeal

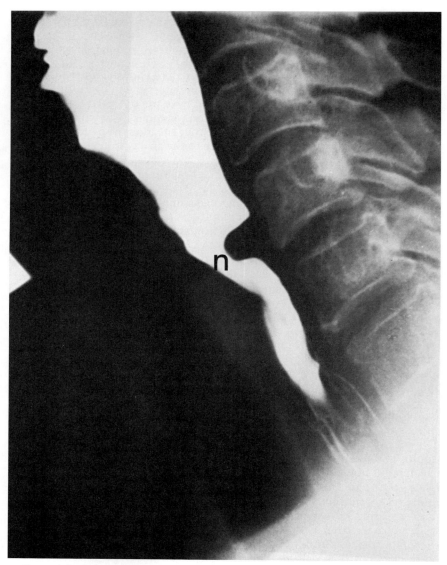

FIGURE 6-1 The cricopharyngeal muscle has pushed into the barium column, causing a narrowing (*n*) of the barium column. This creates the visual impression of a "bar."

spasm; however, the narrowing does not result in a temporary obstruction to flow. Rather, it results in a permanent obstruction. The stenosis is unyielding and is present during swallowing and nonswallowing acts. This type of stenosis is an **anatomic stenosis,** to be distinguished from a physiologic stenosis. An example of an anatomic stenosis can be viewed in the videotape that accompanies this text (Crary and Groher, *Video Introduction to Adult Swallowing Disorders,* Butterworth-Heinemann).

Zenker's Diverticulum. A Zenker's diverticulum is a pouch that develops in the hypopharynx that results in the accumulation of food and fluid. The presence of the pouch interferes with normal bolus flow through the PES. Patients often complain of food sticking in the neck with regurgitation and halitosis. The etiologies of the diverticulum formation are not well known. Because a Zenker's diverticulum typically forms at the junction of the oblique and circular fibers of the hypopharynx (Killian's dehiscence, Figure 2-4), and because a Zenker's diverticulum is seen most often in older persons, some authors have speculated that the diverticulum develops simply because a person has swallowed for many years. Resulting muscle weakness causes the pouch to form into a space of least resistance. Autopsy analysis of the cricopharyngeal muscle of persons with Zenker's diverticulum supports the notion of muscle degeneration similar to that seen in other striated muscles in older persons. Other investigators have noted the high incidence of GERD in patients with Zenker's diverticulum and have speculated that GERD may be a causative factor. One theory is that GERD precipitates esophageal motility disorders that result in abnormal swallowing pressures exerted on the region of the PES. The response to these abnormal pressures is the formation of a pouch (Zenker's diverticulum). An example of Zenker's diverticulum pouch can be seen in Figure 6-2.

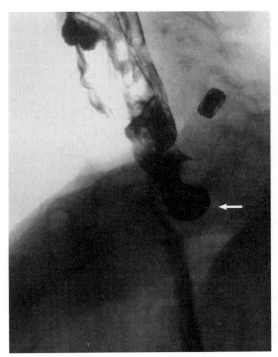

FIGURE 6-2 Example of a Zenker's diverticulum. Note the pouchlike effect with barium collection.

PES Webs. A web is a small piece of tissue or membrane that extends across a lumen, causing it to narrow. Webs can be found in the cervical region and in the esophagus. When webs are well formed, they can cause dysphagic symptoms. The causative mechanisms for web formation are speculative but include increased pressure on the pharynx from poor esophageal motility and GERD. Unless the examiner uses slow motion in radiographic interpretation, some webs will not be detected.

GERD and the Larynx

Acid that is refluxed through the PES may burn the mucosa of the laryngeal structures. Severe inflammation may precipitate dysphagia. Symptoms of globus, odynophagia, vocal disorders including **granuloma**, generalized airway protection problems (poor laryngeal reflex response including laryngospasm), laryngeal stenosis, and cancer have been described. All of these disorders may be associated with dysphagia. Interference with the normal opening and closing of the laryngeal valve may result in airway protection mechanics during the moment of swallow. If acid is allowed to seep below the level of the true vocal folds, respiratory injury may result. Such injury could compromise the laryngeal valve by altering respiratory patterns from lung compromise, making it difficult to keep the airway closed during a swallowing sequence. Changes in respiratory rate or capacities also may make it difficult to apply enough expiratory force after the swallow to clear penetrated material from the vocal folds.

GERD and the Mouth

Few patients with GERD complain that acid reaches the level of the oral cavity. However, in addition to the acrid taste, patients with this complaint also show signs of dental enamel erosion and inflammation. Both may result in odynophagia and difficulty in bolus preparation.

TAKE HOME NOTES

- Patients whose swallowing disorder is localized to the region of the PES may have a primary abnormality in the PES or may have a secondary abnormality in the PES resulting from primary esophageal disease.
- GERD may impact swallowing by direct contact of acid on the aerodigestive tract mucosa and by irritation to the vagal complex, which controls swallowing and related (respiratory) behaviors.
- GERD can potentially be a causative factor in swallowing disorders that involve the entire aerodigestive tract.
- Disorders of the PES without a clear cause include fibrosis, cricopharyngeal bar or spasm, and Zenker's diverticulum.

CASE EXAMPLE

A 40-year-old man came to the clinic with the complaint that solid food was sticking in his throat for the past year. He reported that he had a significant history of

GERD and was taking **proton-pump inhibitors** irregularly. He noted that he had lost 10 pounds in the last 3 months. A videofluorographic swallowing study revealed a hypertrophic cricopharyngeal muscle that caused a reduction in the flow of solid food through the region of the PES. However, the solid-food bolus did enter the esophagus and did not spill into the airway. Because the obstruction to solid food was not judged as severe, and because the patient had a history of GERD that had not been reeval-uated, a standard barium esophagram was ordered. This study revealed a significant narrowing in the region of the LES with abnormal esophageal motility and a dilated esophagus. It was suggested that the patient be referred to a gastroen-terologist for esophageal endoscopy. Endoscopy revealed marked esophageal stenosis at the junction of the esophagus and stomach.

In this case, the patient's complaint of solid food sticking in the neck was veri-fied by the videofluorographic swallowing study. However, the history suggested that the patient had suffered a significant amount of weight loss. The amount of weight loss seemed disproportionate to the degree of PES narrowing. In addition, the patient had a history of GERD that probably was not well controlled. Because of his history, he was prone to primary esophageal disease, and tests confirmed this suspicion. The abnormality seen in the PES was probably a result of excessive pres-sure changes put on the PES from a lack of esophageal motility. Alternative hypotheses for PES dysfunction include direct acid contact that resulted in cricopharyngeal hypertrophy or an irritation of CN X that resulted in poor PES opening and closing mechanics. Treatment in this case was aimed at dilation of the LES stricture and medication to control the GERD.

CHAPTER TERMS

anatomic stenosis constant, nonyielding narrowing of a lumen

Barrett's esophagus inflammation and ulceration of the lower esophageal sphincter caused by gastroesophageal reflux disease; usually considered a precancerous condition

dysplasia abnormal changes in or development of tissue

edema swelling

fibrosis formation of scar tissue in place of normal connective tissue that may result in muscle immobility

granuloma a growth that develops when the immune system cannot fight off an inflammatory process

muscle hypertrophy an increase in the size of a muscle caused by excessive functional activity or as compensation to irritation

physiologic stenosis temporary narrowing of a lumen that eventually opens

pneumonitis inflammation of the lungs

proton-pump inhibitors a class of drugs used to reduce the production of stomach acid

SUGGESTED READINGS

Cruse JP et al: The pathology of cricopharyngeal disease, *Histopathology* 3:223, 1979.

Demeester TR et al: Chronic respiratory symptoms and occult gastrointestinal reflux, *Ann Surg* 211:337, 1990.

Holloway RH: Abnormalities of esophageal body response to distension in reflux disease, *Am J Med* 103:47S, 1997.

Jones B et al: Pharyngoesophageal interrelationships: observations and working concepts, *Gastrointest Radiol* 10:225, 1985.

Kilman WJ, Goyal RK: Disorders of pharyngeal and upper esophageal sphincter motor function, *Arch Intern Med* 136:592, 1976.

Lazarchik DA, Filler SJ: Effects of gastroesophageal reflux on the oral cavity, *Am J Med* 103:107S, 1997.

Pearlman NW, Steigmann GV, Teter A: Primary upper aerodigestive tract manifestations of gastroesophageal reflux, *Am J Gastroenterol* 83:22, 1988.

Sivit CJ et al: Pharyngeal swallow in gastroesophageal reflux disease, *Dysphagia* 2:151, 1988.

Spechler SJ, Goyal RK: Barrett's esophagus, *N Engl J Med* 315:362, 1986.

Stein M et al: Cricopharyngeal dysfunction in chronic obstructive pulmonary disease, *Chest* 97:347, 1990.

Toohill RJ, Kuhn JC: Role of refluxed acid in pathogenesis of laryngeal disorders, *Am J Med* 103:100S, 1997.

CHAPTER 7

Physical Evaluation

FOCUS QUESTIONS

1 What is the rationale for performing a clinical evaluation for a swallowing disorder?
2 Discuss some of the key components from the medical history that might be important in defining the cause of dysphagia.
3 What are the key components to the physical evaluation of the swallowing mechanism?
4 Are there standardized tests that evaluate the clinical aspects of swallowing performance?

RATIONALE

The physical evaluation of the patient with dysphagia has three main components: the medical history, the physical inspection of the swallowing musculature, and observations of swallowing competence with test swallows. Logemann lists five reasons for performing a clinical (physical) evaluation for a swallowing disorder: (1) to define a potential cause (medical history), (2) to establish a working hypothesis that defines the disorder, (3) to establish a tentative treatment plan, (4) to develop a potential list of questions that may need further study, and (5) to establish the patient's readiness to cooperate with any further testing. For reasons of patient cooperation or performance, not all elements of the physical evaluation may be completed. In this circumstance, the clinician has to rely heavily on the medical history or, if the patient is eating, on observations of his or her swallowing ability.

MEDICAL HISTORY

The medical history can be assembled from prior or current medical records, from conversations with the medical staff if the patient is hospitalized, and verbally from the patient or family. Conversations with the patient often are needed to supply missing data or to elucidate or confirm unclear data. If the patient's mental status is not compromised, the physical examination often begins with the patient describing his or her dysphagic symptoms. This description can be useful in developing specific areas of emphasis during the physical and laboratory evaluation. Chapter 3 details the importance of symptom complaints and should be reviewed in conjunction with this chapter.

Elements

A sample medical history form is presented in Figure 7-1. It can be used to guide the examiner in gathering important historical elements that may

101

Patient's name:_____

Date of birth:_____

Gender:_____

Medical record number:_____

Chief complaint:_____

_____

_____

Source of information:

___Patient

___Family

___Recent medical record

___Past history

___Other source

Congenital Family Illness:

   Neurologic disease:

      ___Stroke

      ___Progressive disease

      ___Traumatic injury

      ___Other CNS disorders

      ___Medications taken for:

   Psychiatric disease:

      ___Medications taken for:

      ___Movement disorder

   Surgical procedures:

      ___Spinal fusion

      ___Myotomy

      ___Alimentary tract

FIGURE 7-1 Sample medical history form.

___Fundoplication

___Head/neck cancer

___Thyroidectomy

___Cardiac

Cancer-related:

___Irradiation

___Chemotherapy

Systemic/metabolic:

___Nutrition/hydration status

___Current and ideal weight

___Laboratory values related to nutrition

___Infections

___Toxins

___Diabetes

Respiratory Impairment:

___Chronic obstructive pulmonary disease

___Prior history of aspiration pneumonia

___Cardiopulmonary disease

Esophageal Disease:

___Reflux/regurgitation

___Motility disorder

___Dilatation

Prior test results:

___Radiographic

___Manometric

___Scintigraphic

___Endoscopic

Current Advance Directive Status:_____

FIGURE 7-1 Cont'd.
For legend see opposite page.

impact the diagnosis and treatment of a person with dysphagia. This information can be obtained from the patient, the caregiver, or the medical record. Some patients, such as those who suffered a stroke and have dysphagia, make the connection between their neurologic impairment and their complaint. However, others, such as those who have dysphagia following stomach surgery, may not make the connection between their surgery and dysphagia. For example, in patients who have had stomach surgery, the dysphagia may be related more to the **endotracheal tube** placed in the airway during surgery than to any disorder in the stomach. Therefore it is important to take a complete inventory of the patient's medical history.

The medical history as presented in Figure 7-1 is divided into 10 parts: congenital disease, neurologic disease, psychiatric disease, surgical procedures, cancer-related procedures, metabolic disorders, respiratory impairment, esophageal disorders, prior evaluations of swallowing, and the patient's **Advance Directive** status.

Congenital Disease. Disorders from childhood, particularly those with neurogenic origin such as cerebral palsy, should be noted. These disorders may not have resulted in dysphagia in the past, but may have more significance relative to the present complaint.

Neurologic Disease. Neurologic disorders are the most common cause of dysphagia. Stroke, head trauma, and progressive neurogenic diseases such as multiple sclerosis, amyotrophic lateral sclerosis, and Parkinson's disease often precipitate dysphagia. (For a full discussion of neurologic swallowing disorders, see Chapter 4.) It is important to note any medical complications from the disease and, in particular, any side effects from medications that may be taken to control the disease but that may have adverse effects on swallowing. For example, a patient who is taking a central nervous system depressant to control seizures may have a concomitant depression in motor function that affects swallowing.

Surgical Procedures. Any surgical procedure has the potential to create dysphagic symptoms, particularly if the patient underwent general anesthesia that required the placement of an endotracheal tube through the vocal folds. Damage to the vocal folds can interfere with airway protection, resulting in dysphagia. Any surgical procedure that involves the aerodigestive or respiratory tract should be noted. Patients who have undergone a surgical wrap **(fundoplication)** of the lower esophageal sphincter to control gastroesophageal reflux disease may be dysphagic because the wrap is too tight. Patients who have undergone surgical relaxation **(myotomy)** of the upper or lower esophageal sphincter should have the circumstances of the outcome explored (e.g., Did it help their swallowing disorders?). Surgery to control cancer in the head, neck, and esophagus is of particular importance. Noting whether the cancer also was treated by chemotherapy or radiation therapy may help explain common side effects from those therapies that may cause dysphagia. Other specific surgical procedures to note include cardiopulmonary surgery, thyroid surgery, surgery in the upper airway, and cervical spine surgery. The risk in these procedures of damaging cranial nerve (CN) X is higher than in other surgical procedures in these regions, and therefore places the patient at greater risk for dysphagia.

Systemic and Metabolic Disorders. Disturbances in the body's chemical balance that result from toxins (secondary to medication intolerance) or infections may act secondarily on the central nervous system, resulting in symptoms of dysphagia. Disorders of metabolism may result in dehydration and undernutrition, compromising physical and mental performance. Physical weakness and mental confusion can be precursors to the dysphagic condition. Asking the patient to comment on any recent weight loss or to compare his or her current weight with prior weight may provide insight into the severity of the patient's dysphagia. Diabetes is an example of a systemic, metabolic disorder that may affect swallowing, particularly esophageal peristalsis.

Respiratory Impairment. Because respiration and deglutition share common interactions, any compromise to the respiratory system may decompensate swallowing. Therefore it is important to ask patients whether they have any respiratory disease such as chronic obstructive pulmonary disease or asthma in their medical history. Patients who report being treated for suspected aspiration pneumonia already have shown signs of an inability to adequately protect the airway.

Esophageal Disease. Problems with esophageal motility or with stenosis of the esophageal body can provide important clues in defining the dysphagic condition. Some patients may have a history of an enlarged heart that could be compressing the esophagus. Others may have a history of regurgitation or reflux that has required treatment such as dilation. If a patient has received specialized treatment or tests in the esophagus, the response to that treatment should be noted.

Prior Test Results. Any laboratory study, such as endoscopy of the upper airway, esophagus, or stomach, should be explored. The results of any radiographic studies, such as a barium swallow, a modified barium swallow, or an ultrasound of the aerodigestive tract, are of interest. Some patients with dysphagia and reflux may have undergone a scintigraphic evaluation in nuclear medicine to define the amount and extent of their reflux. Other patients may have undergone a 24-hour pH study to evaluate the presence and frequency of reflux.

Advance Directive. A patient may or may not have executed an Advance Directive stating his or her preference about tube feeding if dysphagia is severe. If an Advance Directive has been executed and is part of the medical record, it should be reviewed. If the patient has chosen not to be tube fed under any circumstances, the need for further testing or treatment may be contraindicated.

PHYSICAL EXAMINATION

The physical examination specific to swallowing impairment typically includes observations of medical interventions that may affect swallowing, such as a tracheostomy tube, and assessment of the patient's mental status and of the cranial nerves involved in swallowing. If the patient is eating, observations of his or her swallowing and feeding skills during test swallow attempts

| **Box 7-1** | *Guidelines for the Clinical Evaluation of Swallowing* |

Clinical Observations
Feeding method
- Nasogastric
- Gastrostomy
- Jejunostomy
- Intravenous

Respiratory status
- SpO$_2$ level
- Tracheostomy
- Ventilator
- Rate

Mental status
- Level of alertness
- Orientation
- Cooperation
- Sustained attention

Cognitive screening
- Memory
- Language
- Perception

Cranial Nerve Assessment
CN V
- Jaw opening and closing
- Jaw lateralization
- Muscle strength, bite down

CN VII
- Facial muscles at rest
- Pucker, smile
- Raise eyebrow
- Lips closed against resistance

CN IX, X
- Gag reflex
- Velum
- Voice
- Cough
- Dry swallow

CN XII
- Tongue range of motion
- Tongue strength
- Fasciculations, atrophy

Oral Cavity Inspection
- Lesions, thrush
- Moisture
- Dentition

Test Swallows
- Thin liquid
- Thick liquid
- Pudding consistency
- Semisolid

Cervical auscultation results
- Normal sounds
- Abnormal sounds
- Swallow delay
- Respiratory changes

Mealtime Observations
- Posture
- Ambiance
- Self-feeding skills
- Utensil use
- Assistance needed
- Diet level
- Respiratory pattern changes

are made. A checklist of items of interest in the clinical evaluation of the dysphagic patient is presented in Box 7-1.

Investigators have sought to determine which elements in the clinical examination for swallow are important in detecting and defining the disorder. Research evidence supports the importance of the following elements: dysphonia (harshness and breathiness), a wet-sounding voice, dysarthria, secretion management, a volitional cough, and laryngeal elevation. The finding of two or more of these clinical markers after clinical examination was more predictive of dysphagia and an unsafe swallow than the finding of only a single feature.

One investigation found that in acute stroke patients, the clinical examination of swallowing, when compared with videofluoroscopic examination, underestimated the detection of dysphagia but overestimated the frequency of aspiration. During trials, the most important elements include failure to swallow thin liquids, a wet voice after swallow, failure to swallow thick liquids, a cough after swallow, and a lack of ability to self-feed.

Clinical Observations

A portion of the physical examination can be completed with basic observations of the patient's medical status. These observations are particularly important for patients who are bedfast and undergoing medical or surgical treatment. Some assumptions can be made about swallowing performance based on observational data.

Feeding Tubes. Some patients may not be eating orally or may be taking part of their nutrition through a feeding tube. A nasogastric tube that is inserted through the nose and into the stomach is easily visible (Figure 7-2A). Feeding tubes come in various sizes. Larger ones may be needed to pass medications without clogging. Smaller, more flexible ones, called *Dobhoff™ tubes*, provide more comfort to the patient. Evidence suggests that the presence of a feeding tube through the nose may slow the sequence of the pharyngeal swallow regardless of the size. Feeding tubes that are placed in the stomach (gastrostomy) or **jejunum** (jejunostomy) may not be visible unless they are connected to a feeding pump (Figure 7-2B). Other patients may be hydrated through intervenous feeding catheters that are placed in the arm and connected to a plastic bag that contains specialized nutrients or medications.

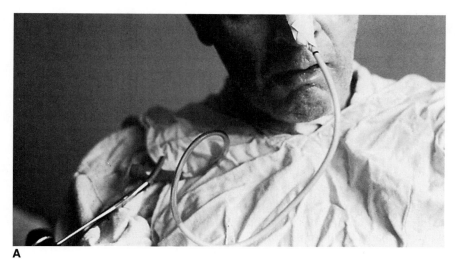

A

FIGURE 7-2 **(A)** A large-bore nasogastric feeding tube is inserted through the left nostril and taped in place. Formula is fed through the end clamped by a hemostat. **(B)** An example of a gastrostomy tube. The patient receives a feeding through the tube that is connected to a bag of formula (bolus delivery) above the level of the patient's head.

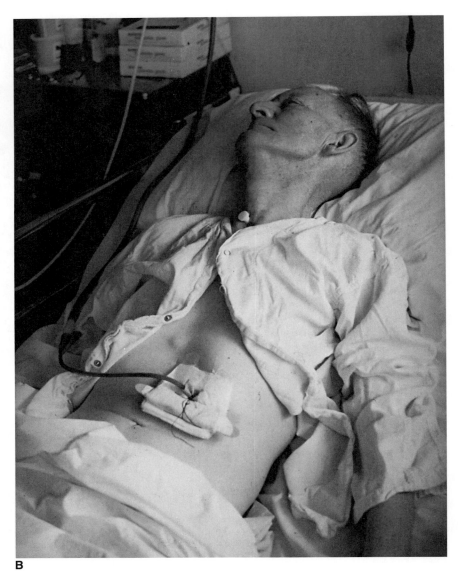

B

FIGURE 7-2 Cont'd.
For legend see previous page.

Tracheostomy Tubes. Tracheostomy tubes are placed when the medical team requires access to the lungs to maintain pulmonary toilet. Often, they are placed when the patient is in respiratory distress or when the upper airway is blocked following trauma or surgery. The size of the tube (in millimeters) is printed on the side. Larger tubes (8 mm) may make it more difficult for the patient to swallow and talk because they block the flow of air to the vocal folds and restrict laryngeal elevation. Smaller-bore (6-mm) tracheostomy tubes allow air to flow past the

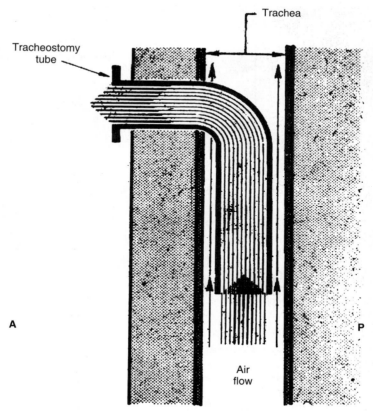

Trachea

Tracheostomy
tube

A

P

Air
flow

FIGURE 7-3 Tracheostomy tube in the trachea below the level of the vocal folds. The lumen of the tracheostomy tube restricts airflow to the level of the vocal folds. *A,* Anterior neck; *P,* posterior neck.

lumen of the tracheostomy tube to vibrate the vocal folds (Figure 7-3). Some tracheostomy tubes come with an inflatable cuff. When the cuff is inflated, the entrance to the trachea is sealed at the level of inflation; however, the patient still can breathe through the lumen of the tracheostomy tube. Theoretically, the cuff is inflated so that the patient's secretions will not flow from the mouth and pharynx into the lungs. The cuff is inflated through a plastic line that rests on the patient's chest. If the bulb on the end of the line is inflated, the cuff in the patient's trachea is inflated. A cuffed tracheostomy tube, inflated and deflated, can be seen in Figure 7-4. Because all types and sizes of tracheostomy tubes may interfere with vocal fold closure and may restrict laryngeal elevation during swallowing, their presence should be noted as part of the clinical evaluation.

Respiratory Pattern. If the patient is bedfast, he or she may be connected to a respirator that assists in the ventilation of the lungs. The ventilator often is connected to a tracheostomy tube with a cuff. The cuff is inflated so that air cannot leak upward from the lungs when the respirator is functioning. When

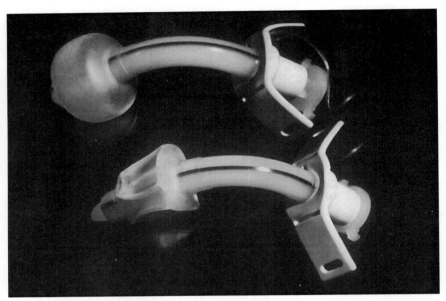

FIGURE 7-4 An example of a cuffed tracheostomy tube. On the *bottom,* the cuff is deflated, on the *top,* it is inflated.

a patient is receiving breathing assistance by a ventilator, swallowing attempts may not be safe. Most clinicians prefer that the medical team partially wean the patient from ventilator support before attempting oral feeding. Observations of the patient's ventilatory pattern can be made by watching the chest rise and fall. Rapid rates (more than 40 cycles/min) make it difficult to close the airway for a sufficient amount of time during the swallow. Some patients' respiration rate and oxygen saturation levels (SpO_2) are measured by sensors attached to their skin. For some patients, oxygen saturation levels (ratio of oxygen to arterial blood) that drop below 90% may indicate a risk for swallowing impairment. Respiratory rates and oxygen saturation levels can be monitored on a screen at the patient's bedside (Figure 7-5). For cooperative patients, a screening of vital and tidal respiratory capacities can be performed in the clinic or at the bedside with a portable respirometer. It has been shown that declining respiratory capacities are predictive of airway protection disorders in patients with amyotrophic lateral sclerosis.

Mental Status. Observations of the bedfast patient may provide a preliminary indicator of mental status. For instance, patients who are alert often respond when the examiner enters the room, either visually by making eye contact or verbally with a greeting. These positive responses allow the examiner to assume that the patient may be able to cooperate with the remainder of the physical examination. Patients who do not easily alert to the examiner's presence or who are unable to sustain attention even after constant encouragement probably are not candidates for safe oral ingestion. Because of the patient's failure to cooperate, the physical examination may be limited. Patients who are uncooperative, either from failure to attend or from extreme agitation, or those who are difficult to arouse should be reexamined periodically during the day. In some cases, the side effects of medications may interfere with normal mental status, whereas in other cases, medications may improve mental status. If the patient is able to cooperate, an assessment of orientation, linguistic skills, perceptual ability, and memory should be made. These learning modalities are important in giving the examiner an impression of the patient's ability to cooperate and learn during

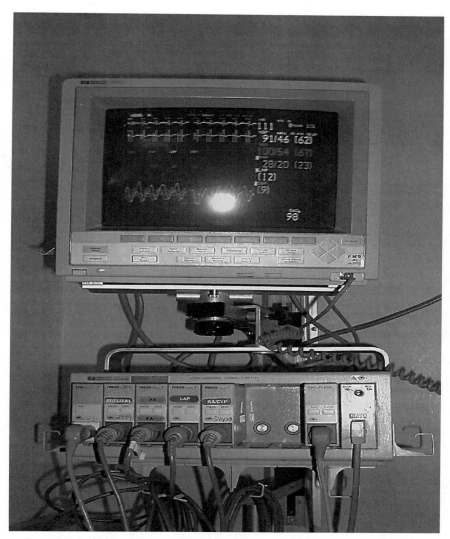

FIGURE 7-5 Bedside monitors track the oxygen saturation level (as a percentage), heart rate, and blood pressure on a single screen. The oxygen saturation level is monitored by a sensor that is attached to the hand or foot. On the lower right corner of this screen, the SpO$_2$ can be read as 98%.

dysphagia treatment. For example, patients who are confused and disoriented may need maximal assistance when eating (for feeding and for reminders of how to perform therapeutic techniques that are needed for their care).

Cranial Nerve Examination

Chapter 2 provides a review of the key cranial nerves involved in swallowing: V, VII, IX, X, XI, and XII. The physical examination of the head and neck musculature for swallowing should focus on gathering information on the function of these cranial nerves. The focus of the examination usually is on the motor aspects of their innervations. The examiner should look for any abnormality, including asymmetry, weakness, abnormal movements at rest, and abnormal movements during volitional efforts.

Facial Muscles. Observations of the facial muscles can be made at rest and during tasks such as lip pursing and smiling. Asking the patient to keep his or her lips closed against the examiner's attempt to pull them apart serves as a test for judging lip strength. The lower and upper facial muscles should be tested to differentiate between **upper and lower motoneuron** damage.

Muscles of Mastication. An assessment of the muscles of mastication begins by having the patient move his or her jaw up and down and laterally. Restrictions in mouth opening **(trismus)** should be noted. The strength of the masticator muscles can be appreciated by palpation as the patient bites down (Figure 7-6).

Tongue Musculature. The examiner should ask the patient to protrude his or her tongue and move it laterally. Rapid tongue movements may be assessed by asking the patient to repeat tongue-tip sounds such as "ta" rapidly. The examiner should then ask the patient to move his or her tongue tip to the roof

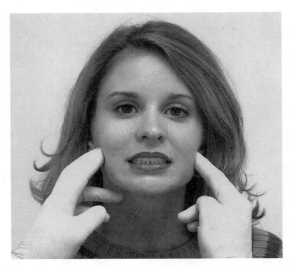

Figure 7-6 Asking the patient to bite down while palpating the response of the masseter muscles provides information about the integrity of the motor function of CN V.

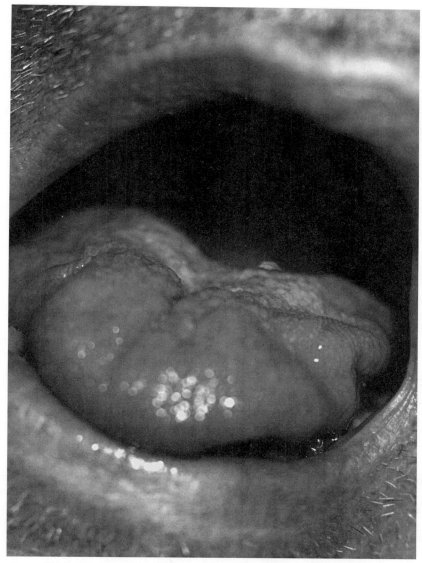

FIGURE 7-7 Lower motoneuron damage is assumed from the significant tongue atrophy (loss of tissue bulk) seen as deep grooves throughout the entire tongue surface.

of the mouth, an activity important during bolus transfer. The protrusion of the patient's tongue against a tongue blade gives the examiner a gross estimate of tongue strength. The tongue should be inspected for atrophy, particularly along the lateral borders. The examiner should look for **fasciculations** if atrophy is seen (Figure 7-7); both are consistent with lower motoneuron

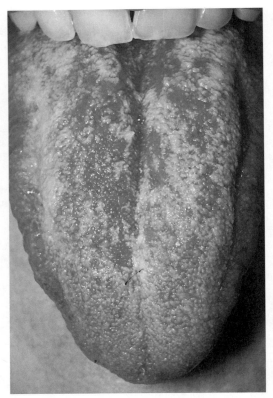

FIGURE 7-8 White-appearing lesions on the tongue are consistent with thrush (oral candidiasis). (From Neville B et al: *Oral and maxillofacial pathology*, ed 2, Philadelphia, 2002, WB Saunders.)

involvement. If the patient's tongue has been resected because of cancer, the amount that has been spared should be noted. The examiner should test sensation with a tongue blade in the region of the reconstruction by asking the patient whether there is a difference between touch in the reconstructed region and in the region that has not been reconstructed. Knowing where the most sensitive area is may be important in food placement during treatment.

Oral Cavity. With the patient's mouth open, the examiner should inspect the oral cavity for any lesions. The milky-white appearance of candidiasis (thrush) is indicative of a fungal infection (Figure 7-8) that if left untreated, may cause **odynophagia**. It is often seen in patients whose immune system has been decompensated by acute or chronic disease. The examiner should check to see whether there is a normal amount of saliva. Patients with **xerostomia** often have little moisture throughout the oral cavity. The tongue may appear reddened and secretions may be thick. Finally, the examiner should inspect the dentition. Teeth in poor repair or ill-fitting dentures may contribute to dysphagia.

Oropharynx. The velum should be observed while at rest and during tasks of phonation. By placing a tongue blade or a gloved finger on the posterior tongue surface of a cooperative patient, the examiner can assess the gag reflex. If the patient has a gag response, it is important to note whether the velum rose and whether the patient elicited a cough. Some patients do not elicit a gag reflex until the tongue base is stimulated. Elicitation of the gag reflex accompanied by a cough provides information about the integrity of CNs IX and X in the oropharynx (velum) and at the level of the larynx (vocal fold closure). The presence of a gag reflex is not an indication that the patient has a normal swallow response. The absence of a gag reflex as an isolated abnormal finding in the examination of the cranial nerves for swallowing may not be important.

Pharynx. There are no tests of pharyngeal function that can be easily appreciated during the physical evaluation of the swallowing response. In some patients, the activity of the superior pharyngeal constrictor muscle can be observed after an active gag reflex or during the production of a falsetto voice. The activity of the pharyngeal constrictor muscles is best visualized by endoscopy.

Larynx. Asking the patient to phonate or listening to his or her vocal quality in conversation provides useful information on the integrity of the airway protective mechanism. Hoarseness and breathiness, as well as a wet, gurgling-sounding voice, are laryngeal abnormalities associated with dysphagia and difficulty protecting the airway. Asking the patient to produce a "dry" swallow while palpating the larynx at the level of the thyroid notch (Figure 7-9) helps the examiner assess the presence and extent of laryngeal elevation. Normal elevation ranges from 2 to 4 cm.

Test Swallows

In a cooperative, alert patient who, up to this point in the examination, has not demonstrated significant neurologic impairment and who has been able to swallow his or her own secretions without significant airway compromise, the examiner may want to grossly assess the swallow response using real food items. Most examiners use an array of items, ranging from thin to thickened liquids, to pudding and softer items, to items that require mastication. Volumes usually range from 5 to 10 ml, starting first with a smaller-size bolus and, if successful, moving toward larger boluses. If successful on 10-ml boluses, the examiner may wish to test the swallow with a 20-ml bolus. The clinician should make observations of chewing and bolus preparation. One clinical method of making a judgment of whether the swallow response is delayed is the use of cervical auscultation. The examiner places a stethoscope on the neck at the level of the vocal folds and listens for the sounds that are associated with swallowing (Figure 7-10). Before the swallow, the examiner notes the respiratory rate. Comparisons should be made between the predeglutitory respiration pattern and the postdeglutitory respiratory pattern. Significant change in rate or an increase in respiratory congestion may be a sign of airway compromise. During swallow, respirations should cease (period of apnea). Within the short apneic period, two bursts of sound are markers of the presence of a swallow. These can be heard by cervical auscultation. Studies of

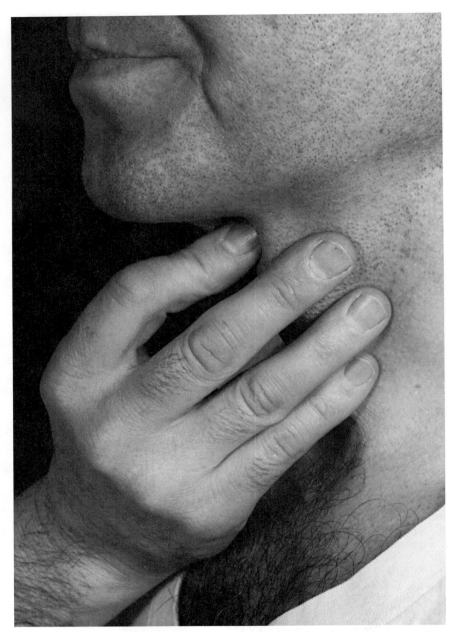

FIGURE 7-9 The examiner palpates at the level of the thyroid notch to feel for laryngeal elevation as a sign that a swallow response has been elicited.

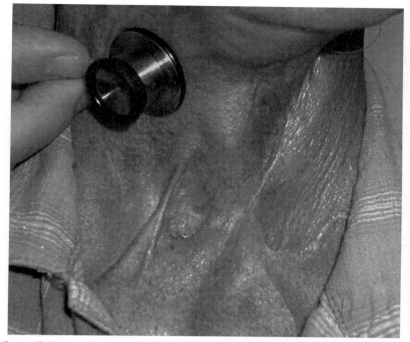

FIGURE 7-10 A stethoscope placed on the side of the neck can provide important acoustic information about the swallow response.

simultaneous videofluoroscopy and swallowing sounds have shown that the first burst of sound is associated with the bolus content that has entered the pharynx, whereas the second sound is associated with the bolus as it leaves the pharynx and enters the esophagus (Figure 7-11).

After most normal swallows, a short exhalation can be heard as a single short burst of acoustic energy. Detecting a delay in these sounds, or failure to hear any of these sounds, may serve as potential markers of swallow abnormality. An acoustic representation of an entire respiratory-swallowing sequence is presented in Figure 7-12.

Feeding Evaluation

Patients who are unable to cooperate with a physical evaluation and who may be eating with suspected dysphagic complications can be partially evaluated through careful observation at the bedside. Bedside data should be gathered for three meals, because the eating circumstance, including differing food items, may vary from breakfast to lunch to dinner.

Environment. Patients with cortical brain damage and dysphagia may be highly distractible. If the distraction causes the patient to talk while eating or not to focus on the process of feeding, swallowing safety may be sacrificed. Typical distractions include the radio, the television, and the feeding assistant

Bolus Entry

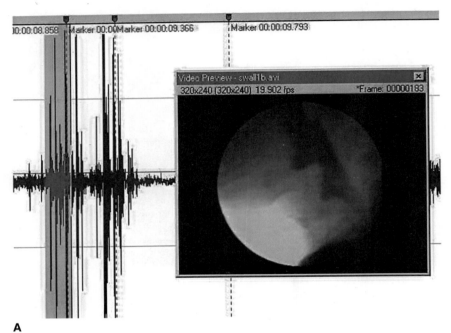

A

FIGURE 7-11 **(A)** Simultaneous recording of the videofluoroscopic image of swallow and the corresponding acoustic pattern. The first swallow sound burst is associated with the bolus entry into the pharynx. **(B)** The second sound burst should be associated with the bolus leaving the pharynx and entering the esophagus. (Courtesy T. Neil McKaig.)

asking the patient for a verbal response while eating. Other distractions include those that are patient centered; for example, the patient's glasses are not positioned properly, resulting in distraction, or his or her attention is focused on an ill-fitting denture that is causing discomfort.

Feeding. If the patient is self-feeding, the clinician must answer the following questions: Is he or she able to open all containers, to find the food on the tray, and to use the utensils properly? Is he or she able to use the utensils to transport food to the mouth? Is the feeding rate appropriate? Are his or her bite sizes appropriate? Are there differences in swallowing performance between taking liquids using a straw and taking them by cup? If the patient is to use special feeding utensils, are they provided? If the patient needs dentures, are the dentures in place and properly fitted?

Posture. Because an upright posture is best for swallowing, it is important to note whether the patient is in an upright position and whether he or she can maintain that position throughout the meal. If the patient is to use a special posture such as chin down as a method of airway protection, (see Chapter 9)

Bolus Exit

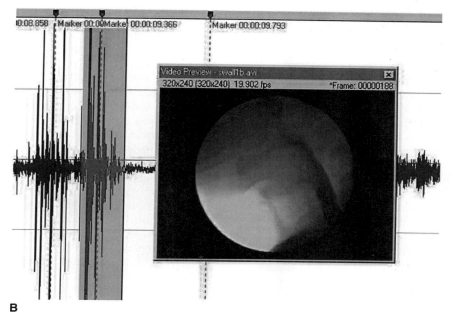

FIGURE 7-11 Cont'd.
For legend see opposite page.

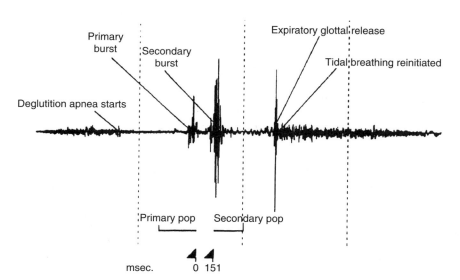

FIGURE 7-12 An acoustic representation of a normal swallow sequence. It is marked by the cessation of tidal airflow and two bursts of swallowing sounds within the apneic period (*first* and *last dotted lines*), followed by a burst of exhalation and the resumption of tidal breathing. (Courtesy T. Neil McKaig.)

observations of whether he or she can achieve this posture should be made. Even in patients who are tube fed by gastrostomy, the head of the bed should be elevated slightly to avoid the possibility of reflux from the stomach.

Eating. The patient's diet level (soft, pureed, mechanical soft, or regular) should be noted. Some patients receive a diet level that is not appropriately matched to their disorder. The clinician must assess whether the consistency of fluids is appropriate if they are to be altered by thickening. If thickened fluids are allowed to sit too long before being served, they may become too thick for safe ingestion. Regarding the patient's diet level, the examiner must pose the following questions: Does the patient have more difficulty with liquids than with semisolids, or visa versa? When the patient places an item that requires mastication in the mouth, does he or she display adequate chewing motion, or does the item sit without the patient making any apparent attempt to start a swallow? Does the patient have choking episodes, either before he or she tries to swallow, during the swallow, or after the swallow has been completed? The use of cervical auscultation or observations of laryngeal elevation may assist the examiner in this determination. The examiner should make observations regarding whether the eating process is more efficient at the beginning or end of the meal, because fatigue may decompensate safe swallowing in some patients. Estimates of the amount eaten and the total time taken to finish the meal are important markers of swallowing efficiency. Changes in respiratory status taken from bedside monitors (SpO_2) or from audible respiratory distress, such as wheezing or difficulty clearing secretions, should be part of the observational data pool.

Assistance. If prior recommendations to improve the patient's feeding or eating performance have been made, the examiner must assess whether the patient is following these suggestions. If the patient is in need of a feeding assistant who must provide reminders to accomplish safe feeding, the examiner must determine whether those reminders are being provided.

FORMALIZED CLINICAL TESTS

Until recently, most clinicians designed their own clinical swallowing evaluation based on the elements they believed were most useful in detecting and defining the dysphagic condition. Most tests were scored with a plus-minus system, and none were psychometrically rigorous. *The Bedside Assessment of Swallowing Safety* was the first computer-based test to regularize the clinical evaluation. It requires the examiner to assign scores to various physical parameters and summarizes those data in a report. The format assists the clinician in setting treatment goals and in determining whether further laboratory testing is warranted.

The Mann Assessment of Swallowing Ability is the first clinical test of swallowing that has psychometric integrity. It has reported reliability and validity data on a population of 128 first-time poststroke patients. It allows the examiner to make judgments of dysphagia and aspiration severity by using clinical diagnostic criteria (an ordinal risk rating) or by adding individual subtest scores and comparing them with the study sample. Scoring guidelines are provided in the following 24 areas of assessment: alertness, cooperation, auditory comprehension, respiration, respiration rate after swallow, aphasia, apraxia, dysarthria, saliva management, lip seal, tongue movement, tongue strength, tongue coordination, oral preparation, gag reflex, palatal movement, bolus clearance, oral transit, cough reflex, voluntary cough, voice, tracheostomy, pharyngeal phase, and pharyngeal response.

TAKE HOME NOTES

- The clinical examination for swallowing has three main components: medical history, physical evaluation, and test swallows.
- The following are five reasons to perform a physical evaluation for swallowing: to define a potential cause for the problem, to establish a working hypothesis to define the disorder, to establish a tentative treatment plan, to develop questions for further study or referral, and to establish the readiness to cooperate with further testing.
- For patients who are eating but who are uncooperative with the physical evaluation, the examiner has to rely on the medical history and on mealtime observations.
- Most of the physical evaluation relies on the assessment of the patient's mental status and on an assessment of the integrity of the cranial nerves.
- *The Mann Assessment of Swallowing Ability* is a standardized clinical test that measures swallowing skills.

CASE EXAMPLE

An elderly woman came into the hospital to have her hip replaced. Her past medical history was remarkable for childhood polio, from which she recovered; **hypertension;** and coronary heart disease. Following her surgery, a nurse noted that she was choking on liquids, and a consult was sent to speech pathology.

The physical evaluation revealed that she was alert, oriented, and cooperative. She was able to sustain a cogent conversation while sitting upright in bed. She told the examiner that because she was choking on liquids, they no longer put them on her meal tray, which consisted of a soft, mechanical diet. She was noted to have an intravenous feeding line in her right arm. An evaluation of her oral peripheral speech mechanism revealed generalized weakness of the tongue and lips, more on the right than on the left. Examination of the muscles of mastication was normal. Her oral cavity was xerostomic, and she was **edentulous**. The gag reflex was present, but not brisk. She was able to produce a voluntary cough and swallow response. Normal laryngeal elevation was noted during her dry swallow attempt. Her voice was markedly hoarse, but not breathy. She did not show any signs of dysarthria. During test swallows of 5 ml of thin liquid, she coughed briskly, without delay, as the larynx was elevating. A commercial thickener was added to the thin liquid. During a test swallow with this consistency, the swallow was prompt, without cough or delay. This was repeated with success on 10- and 20-ml boluses.

The patient was then given a spoonful of pudding. This was swallowed without delay or cough. All swallow attempts were monitored with cervical auscultation so that a judgment of whether there was swallowing delay could be made.

In this case, the patient was able to verbally express her difficulty swallowing thin liquids. Her difficulty was noted by the nurses, who reported that she coughed when swallowing thin liquids. Her problem was compensated by adding thickeners to the thin fluid. Failure to protect her airway on thin fluids could have been related to a temporary decompensation of her airway closure reflex related to the endotracheal tube from recent surgery. Airway closure problems commonly are most obvious when thinner fluids are being swallowed, because of their speed of movement through the pharynx. This possibility was supported by her severe hoarseness. An alternative explanation might be that she had suffered generalized weakness in the bulbar musculature from her childhood polio, which became more apparent at the laryngeal level following her surgery. That muscle weakness still was present was supported by diminished strength in the lip and tongue musculature. Her xerostomia was secondary to side effects from medications taken to control her coronary artery disease. The patient was placed on thickened liquids with a soft mechanical diet. The recommendation to discontinue her intravenous fluids was made, because it was believed that she could maintain hydration with thickened liquids. The prognosis for returning to regular fluids was judged to be good, because it was thought that the decompensation of her airway closure would be temporary. Continued monitoring of her respiratory status was recommended to ensure that she was safe on this dietary level. Because her complaint was explained and ultimately solved by the clinical evaluation, no further testing was considered.

CHAPTER TERMS

Advance Directive a legal document, prepared by a competent individual, that is a statement to guide the health care team in specific medical circumstances, such as whether the person wants a permanent feeding tube

endentulous without teeth

endotracheal tube a tube placed through the mouth and vocal folds to help a patient breathe

fasciculations small muscle fiber twitching often seen in patients with lower motoneuron disease

fundoplication a surgical procedure performed to narrow the opening of the lower esophageal sphincter to prevent gastric reflux

hypertension high blood pressure

jejunum a portion of the small intestine

myotomy surgical relaxation of a group of muscles

odynophagia painful swallowing

trismus restriction in the ability to open the jaw

upper and lower motoneurons the two major divisions of the pyramidal motor tracts: the upper motoneuron governs voluntary movement, and the lower motoneuron governs reflexive movement

xerostomia dryness, particularly in the mouth

SUGGESTED READINGS

Daniels SK et al: Clinical predictors of dysphagia and aspiration risk: outcome measures in acute stroke patients, *Arch Phys Med Rehabil* 81:1030, 2000.

Daniels SK et al: Clinical assessment of swallowing and prediction of dysphagia severity, *Am J Speech Lang Pathol* 6:17, 1997.

Dikeman KJ, Kazandjian MS: *Communication and swallowing management of tracheotomized and ventilator-dependent adults,* San Diego, 1995, Singular Publishing Group.

Groher ME: The case history. In Mills RH, editor: *Evaluation of dysphagia in adults,* Austin, Tx, 2000, Pro-ed.

Horner J et al: Aspiration following stroke: clinical correlates and outcome, *Neurology* 38:1359, 1988.

Huggins PS, Tuomi SK, Young C: Effects of nasogastric tubes on the young, normal swallowing mechanism, *Dysphagia* 14:157, 1999.

Langmore SE, Logemann JA: After the clinical bedside swallowing examination: what next? *Am J Speech Lang Pathol* 1:13, 1991.

Linden P, Kuhlemeier KV, Patterson C: Probability of correctly predicting subglottic penetration from clinical observations, *Dysphagia* 8:170, 1993.

Logemann JA, Veis S, Colangelo L: A screening procedure for oropharyngeal dysphagia, *Dysphagia* 14:44, 1999.

Mann G: *The Mann assessment of swallowing ability,* San Diego, 2001, Singular.

Mann G, Hankey GJ, Cameron D: Swallowing disorders following acute stroke: prevalence and diagnostic accuracy, *Cerebrovasc Dis* 10:380, 2000.

McCullough GH et al: Clinicians' preferences and practices in conducting clinical/ bedside and videofluoroscopic swallowing examinations in an adult, neurogenic population, *Am J Speech Lang Pathol* 8:149, 1999.

McCullough GH et al: Inter- and intra-judge reliability of a clinical examination of swallowing in adults, *Dysphagia* 15:58, 2000.

McKaig TN, Thibodeau J: *The bedside assessment of swallowing safety,* Woburn, Mass, 1998, Butterworth-Heinemann.

Yorkston KA, Miller RM, Strand EA: *Management of speech and swallowing disorders in degenerative disease,* Tucson, Ariz, 1995, Communication Skill Builders.

Instrumental Exam (VIFL + FEES.)

C H A P T E R 8

Instrumental Swallowing Examinations: Fluoroscopy and Endoscopy

FOCUS QUESTIONS

1   Why is it important to "image" the swallowing mechanism and function with an instrumental study? What are some basic guidelines to help determine when any instrumental swallowing examination is indicated?

2   Describe the basic components of a fluoroscopic examination of swallowing function. How might these be modified for various patient groups or swallowing problems? Repeat this process for the endoscopic examination of swallowing function.

3   What are some of the strengths and weaknesses of the fluoroscopic examination of swallowing function? What are some of the strengths and weaknesses of the endoscopic examination of swallowing function?

4   How does the endoscopic examination of swallowing function compare with the fluoroscopic examination specific to the identification of various dysphagia characteristics? What factors might be considered to help in the decision of which instrumental swallowing examination is used?

CONSIDERATIONS FOR AN INSTRUMENTAL SWALLOWING EXAMINATION

Many instrumental procedures may be used to evaluate different aspects of swallowing function. This chapter addresses the two most commonly used procedures: videofluoroscopy (also called *videofluorography*) and flexible endoscopy (also called *fiberoptic endoscopy* or *transnasal endoscopy*). Before these instrumental evaluation procedures are described and discussed, it is important to place them in the context of the overall clinical evaluation of the adult patient with dysphagia. Common questions raised about these procedures include "What are they intended to achieve?" and "When is an instrumental procedure indicated?" The following information comes, in large part, from practice guidelines published by the American Speech-Language Hearing Association (ASHA). The concept behind using practice guidelines is that they result from the creative and clinical input of many experienced professionals with thorough professional review. In that regard, although these views may change with the acquisition of new information, at present, they represent a fair summary of existing knowledge and opinion.

125

Intended Accomplishments of Instrumental Swallowing Evaluations

First, it merits mentioning that instrumental examinations of swallowing are merely a part of the comprehensive examination of swallowing performance and function. In general, a good clinical examination (see Chapter 7) should precede any instrumental examination. The clinical examination can be important in tailoring specific questions to be addressed in an instrumental examination and provides a comprehensive clinical profile of patients with suspected dysphagia. That said, instrumental examinations of swallowing might accomplish any number of objectives depending on the patient and the clinical questions involved. These examinations provide valuable information about the anatomy and physiology of muscles and structures used in swallowing, evaluate the patient's ability to swallow various materials, assess secretions and the patient's reaction to them, document the adequacy of airway protection and the coordination between respiration and swallowing, and help evaluate the impact of compensatory therapy maneuvers on swallowing function and airway protection. The fluoroscopic and endoscopic examinations of swallowing function are not mirror images of each other; however, they do share many common functions, although each adds specific attributes that the other may not possess. Furthermore, because each examination provides a permanent video record of the swallowing examination, both contribute to increased objectivity with enhanced documentation and the ability to review results of the respective studies.

Purposes of Instrumental Swallowing Examinations. Box 8-1 summarizes many purposes attributed to instrumental swallowing examinations. Perhaps the most overt purpose of any instrumental swallowing examination is the

---

Box 8-1   *Multiple Purposes Attributed to an Instrumental Swallowing Study*

- Image structures of the upper aerodigestive tract: oral cavity, velopharynx, pharynx, larynx, pharyngoesophageal segment, esophagus.
- Assess movement patterns of swallowing-related structures in the upper aerodigestive tract to formulate inferences regarding physiologic integrity (e.g., speed of movement, symmetry, range, strength, sensation, coordination).
- Assess swallowing-related movement patterns of structures in the upper aerodigestive tract (e.g., effectiveness and safety of the swallow, accommodation to varying materials).
- Identify and describe any airway compromise (e.g., aspiration, penetration) and the circumstances under which these events occur.
- Evaluate the impact of compensatory maneuvers to improve swallowing safety and efficiency.
- Identify and describe any pooled secretions within the hypopharynx and larynx (or potentially other areas). Description should include the patient's ability to move or clear pooled secretions with swallows or coughing/clearing activities.
- Complete a cursory evaluation of esophageal anatomy and physiology to identify any overt esophageal contributors to dysphagia symptoms.
- Assist in forming clinical recommendations, including route of nutrition or hydration intake (i.e., oral, nonoral), safest or most efficient dietary level, need to make feeding modifications, or therapeutic interventions.

ability to image the structures of the swallowing mechanism and the movement of those structures both during swallowing and during other movements, which may help assess their functional integrity. This assessment involves the lips, tongue, jaw, velopharyngeal mechanism, pharynx, larynx, and esophagus. Evaluation of these structures should incorporate some indication of anatomic adequacy and movement capability. In some cases, it is possible to assess or perhaps infer sensory integrity, as well as motor functions. Beyond basic structure and movement, coordinated movement among various components should be assessed with reference to swallowing function. This requires the patient to swallow materials of varying sizes and textures to permit inspection of adjustments (either positive or negative) within the swallowing mechanism. This component of the instrumental examination can help identify misdirection of a bolus and postswallow residue secondary to inefficient swallowing function. If aspiration is identified, the instrumental examination is helpful in describing those situations in which the patient is more likely to aspirate versus those situations in which the patient is less likely to aspirate. By using a variety of swallowed materials and incorporating compensatory maneuvers, clinicians may make inferences regarding the safest and most efficient material for the patient to swallow and the need for any postural or other adjustments that improve swallowing safety and efficiency. Secretions that are pooled within the swallowing mechanism can be problematic to the patient and can contribute to respiratory complications. These fluids should be identified and described, including the patient's reaction to them and his or her ability to remove them from the swallowing tract. In some situations, it might be concluded that oral feeding is neither safe nor adequate, and hence clinicians might use the results of instrumental examinations to recommend nonoral feeding sources (or in some clinical scenarios, to recommend discontinuation of nonoral feeding sources with reestablishment of oral feeding). In short, instrumental examinations of swallowing function provide objective imaging of the swallowing mechanism, which assists dysphagia clinicians in determining the need for and the direction of swallowing rehabilitation. More details of the fluoroscopic and endoscopic swallowing examinations are provided in the following sections.

Indications for an Instrumental Swallowing Examination

Box 8-2 addresses three important questions: (1) When *is* an instrumental swallowing examination definitely indicated? (2) When *may* an instrumental swallowing examination be indicated? (3) When is an instrumental swallowing examination *not* indicated?

Perhaps the basic answer to when an instrumental examination *is* indicated is when the clinical examination fails to answer the relevant questions. If the patient complains of specific problems that are not clarified by the clinical examination, an instrumental examination is indicated. An instrumental examination may help clarify whether a significant dysphagia exists and what the parameters of that dysphagia are: oral, pharyngeal, esophageal, or a combination of these aspects. Information from an instrumental examination may clarify airway protection issues that are potentially related to respiratory compromise, or it may elucidate swallow efficiency issues potentially related to nutritional decline. As mentioned previously, the impact of compensatory maneuvers may be verified during instrumental examination, and other information on swallowing movements may be garnered that facilitates direction in swallowing rehabilitation.

| **Box 8-2** | *When Is an Instrumental Swallowing Examination Indicated?* |

An Instrumental Swallowing Examination IS Indicated in the Following Circumstances:

- Comprehensive clinical examination fails to thoroughly address the clinical questions posed by the patient and/or problem.
- Dysphagia characteristics are vague and require confirmation or better delineation.
- Nutritional or respiratory issues indicate suspicion of dysphagia.
- Safety or efficiency of swallowing is a concern.
- Direction for swallowing rehabilitation needs to be provided.
- Help is needed to assist in identifying underlying medical problems that contribute to dysphagia symptoms.

An Instrumental Swallowing Examination MAY Be Indicated in the Following Circumstances:

- The patient has a medical condition that has a high risk for dysphagia.
- Swallow function demonstrates an overt change.
- The patient is unable to cooperate for a clinical examination.

An Instrumental Swallowing Examination Is NOT Indicated in the Following Circumstances:

- The patient no longer has dysphagia complaints.
- The patient is too medically compromised or uncooperative to complete the procedure.
- The clinician's judgment is that the examination would not alter the clinical course or management plan.

Finally, in some instances, information gained from an imaging study may contribute to a better understanding of the medical diagnosis that is contributing to the presence of dysphagia symptoms.

An instrumental swallowing examination *may* be indicated for various reasons mostly related to the condition of the patient. For example, some medical conditions pose a high risk for swallowing difficulty or may be complicated by swallowing difficulties that may not merit a significant complaint from the patient. An instrumental examination provides an objective evaluation of swallowing ability that may facilitate early identification of problems and hence lead to improved care. In addition, clinical conditions may change over time either secondary to the underlying disease (i.e., progressing or recovering conditions) or to changes in the patient (new treatments or new disease). Some patients have clinical conditions (e.g., cognitive or communicative impairments) that preclude adequate cooperation with a clinical examination. In these situations, an instrumental examination may help address questions regarding swallowing ability.

Finally, clinical situations exist in which an instrumental examination is *not* indicated. Perhaps the most obvious situation is found with the patient who reports that he or she had difficulty in the past, but no longer experiences any swallowing difficulty. Other situations include patients who are too medically compromised to tolerate a procedure or too uncooperative to participate in a procedure. If the clinician judges that because of the patient's condition, an instrumental examination will provide no useful information, a valid decision may be to delay the examination until the patient's condition facilitates completion of a useful examination. The value of clinical judgment should not be underestimated. At times, clinicians may simply believe that based on all available information, the addition of an instrumental examination of swallowing function will not provide any further beneficial information.

Summary

Instrumental swallowing examinations, specifically the fluoroscopic and endoscopic procedures used to image swallow function, add an objective and valuable component to the comprehensive assessment of the patient with dysphagia. However, these examinations should not be isolated from the information obtained from a thorough clinical assessment. The combination of these tools is expected to provide the most complete clinical picture of the dysphagic patient, leading to the best possible treatment. Instrumental examinations of swallowing function address the anatomy and physiology of structures within the swallowing tract, as well as how movement of these structures accommodates different materials that are swallowed. Clinicians may also assess the impact of immediate compensations with these examinations. Available guidelines offer suggestions for when an instrumental examination should, may, or should not be used; however, no guideline can account for all clinical situations. The judgment of the clinician who has direct knowledge of the comprehensive picture is a valuable tool in deciding when and how to use an instrumental examination of swallowing function.

The following sections address the videofluoroscopic and fiberoptic endoscopic swallowing examinations separately and subsequently compare the two procedures directly to help clinicians decide whether one, both, or neither of these procedures is appropriate in various clinical situations.

VIDEOFLUOROSCOPIC SWALLOWING EXAMINATIONS

Implications of the Name

Various authors and health care institutions use different terms for what is essentially the same examination. Box 8-3 lists several name variants for this procedure. This is not a comprehensive list, but probably representative of the variation that exists in nomenclature. The term *modified barium swallow* can be interpreted literally. The traditional barium swallow is focused on the

---

Box 8-3	*Various Names Used to Describe the Videofluoroscopic Swallowing Study*

- Modified barium swallow (MBS)
- Upper GI series with hypopharynx
- Videofluoroscopic swallow study (VFSS)
- Videofluoroscopic barium examination (VFBE)
- Videofluoroscopic swallow examination (VFSE)
- Rehab swallow study

GI, Gastrointestinal.

esophagus and stomach and uses large amounts of liquid barium **(contrast agent)** and still-frame pictures to image the expanded esophagus and to evaluate gastric emptying or other upper gastrointestinal (GI) functions. This examination is usually performed in one or more combinations of lying positions. The adult patient with dysphagia is likely to be compromised by both the large amounts of liquid barium and the lying position during swallowing attempts. Therefore this examination has been "modified" to use smaller amounts of contrast material varying in size and consistency, and the patient is examined in an upright position (whenever physically possible) to resemble the position most typically associated with eating. This procedure has become known as the *modified barium swallow.*

Some health care professionals and researchers have held to different conventions in selecting a name for this relatively new procedure. GI radiologists often refer to the procedure as an *upper GI series with hypopharynx.* This term reflects the traditional esophagram view but with the addition of a study of the hypopharynx. Other terms in the literature include *videofluorographic swallow study, videofluorographic barium examination,* and even, *videofluorographic swallow examination.* Presumably, each of these terms is intended to identify the unique radiographic procedure that evaluates oropharyngeal swallowing function. In an attempt to reduce confusion within our own health care system, we adopted the term *rehab swallow.* This term, negotiated between the speech-language pathologists and the radiologists, is meant to reflect the importance of this study in *determining the need for and the direction of swallowing rehabilitation.* Inclusion of the word "rehab" helped ensure that a speech-language pathologist was involved in each of these studies that presented to radiology. By performing these studies in conjunction with a radiologist, both the medical and the rehabilitative objectives of this examination were met. Clinicians in different areas may know or use other terms that refer to the same study. In this chapter, the more generic name variant, *videofluoroscopic swallowing examination,* is used.

Objectives of the Videofluoroscopic Swallowing Examination

Many objectives are associated with the videofluoroscopic swallowing examination. The primary objective is to obtain a video image of the upper aerodigestive tract during the act of swallowing. By manipulating what is swallowed, how it is swallowed, and patient positioning, clinicians can complete a comprehensive assessment of swallowing ability. Box 8-4 lists the more overt

---

Box 8-4 *Objectives of the Videofluoroscopic Swallowing Examination*

- Evaluate anatomy and physiology of the swallowing mechanism
- Evaluate swallow physiology
- Identify patterns of impaired swallow physiology
- Identify consequences of impaired swallow physiology
- Evaluate impact of compensations
- Confirm patient symptoms
- Prediction of future functional swallowing performance

objectives of a videofluoroscopic swallowing examination. Additional objectives may be appropriate for individual patients or problems.

Evaluation of the swallowing mechanism is approached initially through identification and description of any deviations in the anatomy of structures within the swallowing tract. This presupposes a detailed knowledge of anatomy, including radiographic anatomy, by the clinician viewing these films. Figure 8-1 depicts both lateral and anterior radiographic views of a normal swallowing mechanism. Review of anatomic detail and both normal and abnormal swallow physiology is found in the video accompanying this text (Crary and Groher, *Video Introduction to Adult Swallowing Disorders*, Butterworth-Heinemann). Physiology of the swallowing mechanism may be evaluated by asking the patient to phonate, breath-hold, perform a Valsalva maneuver, produce falsetto phonation, or perform other activities that facilitate movement of the structures within the swallowing tract. This component of evaluation is helpful in identification of potential movement deficits that may contribute to oropharyngeal dysphagia and in selecting appropriate compensatory maneuvers.

Swallow physiology is evaluated by asking patients to swallow various amounts and textures of contrast materials. Knowledge of both normal and impaired swallow physiology is implicit in evaluating this component of the fluoroscopic examination. Abnormal aspects of physiology typically are detailed in terms of reduced or altered movement patterns. In addition, the consequences of physiologic impairments such as aspiration or residue are documented. Finally, the impact of therapeutic compensations is evaluated. This strategy is useful both for introducing immediate improvement in the safety or efficiency of the swallow and for identifying potentially beneficial therapy strategies.

Symptom confirmation is an important objective of any instrumental examination, including the videofluoroscopic swallowing examination. If a patient complains of food sticking in the lower neck area, the fluoroscopic study should thoroughly evaluate that area. If nothing of consequence is identified in that region, other potential contributors to that symptom should be evaluated (in this specific case, the esophagus and lower esophageal sphincter should be thoroughly evaluated). Addressing symptom confirmation relies heavily on the clinician's skill in focusing the patient's complaints and descriptions of dysphagia symptoms and in directing the fluoroscopic study to adequately evaluate the components of the swallowing mechanism that may contribute to a specific set of symptoms.

Because the fluoroscopic swallowing examination is a time-limited event that cannot possibly sample all foods that a patient might eat, a certain amount of prediction is involved in interpreting this examination. For this reason, *prediction* is included as one of the objectives of the fluoroscopic swallowing examination. After a thorough evaluation of the structure and function of the swallowing mechanism, swallow physiology and consequences of impaired movement, and the impact of compensatory maneuvers, the clinician must engage in a series of educated decisions regarding functional swallowing performance of each patient. Examples of such decisions include the potential for future health complications such as aspiration-related pneumonias and/or nutritional deficits; the level of functional eating ability and any recommended diet-level changes; the need for swallowing therapy; and if

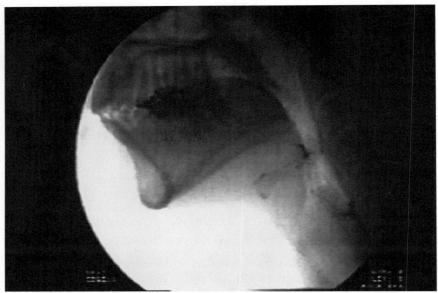

A

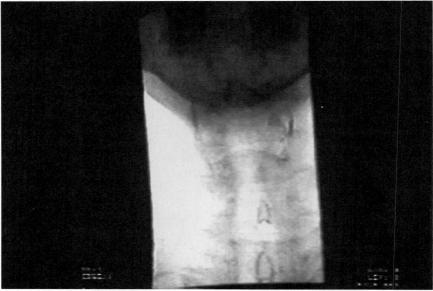

B

FIGURE 8-1 Lateral (**A**) and anterior (**B**) radiographic views of a normal swallowing mechanism.

indicated, the specific direction of that therapy, whether additional clinical or instrumental evaluations are indicated, and whether consults should be sent to other health care providers to address problems identified in the current examination. These are only a few of the potential areas of *prediction* in which clinicians may engage. Ultimately, questions of safe and adequate oral intake of food and liquid must be directly addressed based in part on the results of this examination.

Procedures for the Videofluoroscopic Swallowing Examination

A standard protocol is highly recommended for the fluoroscopic study. Standardizing the protocol increases consistency and reproducibility of examinations both within and across patients. Using a standard protocol does not preclude individual variations that may be required for specific patients or problems; however, it does provide a consistent framework from which reasonable variations may be accomplished. Within the protocol several factors must be considered, including patient positioning, materials to be swallowed, sequence of attempted swallows, and what to look for (including interpretation and documentation of the findings).

Patient Positioning. In large part, positioning depends on the physical abilities of the patient. In general, the videofluoroscopic swallowing examination is accomplished with the patient in an upright, seated position with adequate support for the head and body. Patients who have physical limitations from weakness, fatigue, disease, or other reasons may require special positioning systems during the examination. Various commercial positioning chairs are available to assist in optimal positioning of patients with physical limitations. Before purchasing or building a positioning chair, it is important to know the physical dimensions of the specific fluoroscopic system to be used. Often, there is a fixed maximal distance between the table and the tower of the fluoroscope. In addition, this study typically is completed with both lateral and anterior views. Whichever chair or positioning system is used, it should be adaptable to accommodate both views. Finally, large patients may not fit easily into the fixed space between the table and the tower of the fluoroscope, specifically for lateral views. In this scenario, it is possible to turn the patient slightly toward an oblique orientation while maintaining as much of a lateral perspective as possible.

Typically, this examination begins with the patient in a lateral (or semioblique) position in reference to the fluoroscopic image (Figure 8-2). The lateral perspective affords an excellent view of the swallowing mechanism from lips to cervical esophagus and provides the best view of the trachea separate from the esophagus. This view is beneficial in determining whether material enters the upper airway. Following examination of the swallow in the lateral perspective, the patient is turned for an anterior view. The anterior perspective permits excellent evaluation of symmetry along the swallowing mechanism. When the esophagus is imaged, a sitting position often limits the extent of the view. In these situations, the patient is imaged while standing or in a lying position, depending on the patient's physical limitations or specific aspects of the dysphagia presentation.

Material Used in the Fluoroscopic Study. The key material used in the fluoroscopic study is barium sulfate suspension, which is a positive-contrast agent

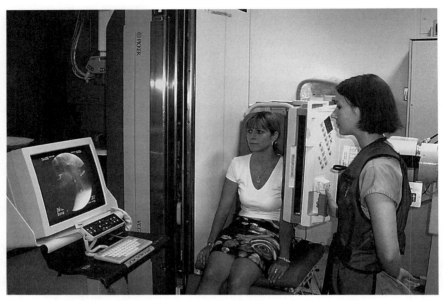

FIGURE 8-2 Patient positioned in fluoroscope for a lateral-view image.

that is **radiopaque.** Thus barium sulfate appears to be black on the fluoroscopic image. This is in comparison with negative-contrast substances, such as air, which appear as varying shades of gray. Tissue and bone appear as shades of gray, depending on their density.

A popular point of discussion and even argument for this study is whether to use barium sulfate in isolation or in combination with real food items. No firm answer has emerged from these discussions, and both perspectives have seemingly valid points. Those individuals who focus on isolated barium products for this study claim that the range of food textures is so vast that it would be impossible to image every possible food or liquid that a patient might ingest. Another argument against using real food is the potential for complications resulting from aspirating food products into the airway. On the converse side of this discussion is the argument that barium products do not represent those consistencies noted in real food products.

Regardless of the outcome of these foods-versus-barium discussions, the importance of using a range of textures and volumes during the fluoroscopic swallowing examination cannot be overstated. It is well known that a normal swallowing mechanism adjusts to changes in bolus size and texture. In the absence of this accommodation, a patient may demonstrate a variety of compensations or demonstrate the consequences of impaired physiology and the inability to compensate. Volumes used in fluoroscopic swallowing studies vary across published reports. One consideration is the average amount ingested by normal-swallowing adults. Published literature suggests that approximately 20 ml of liquid represents the average drink from a cup. An average teaspoon is approximately 5 ml. Therefore it seems reasonable that most swallow attempts would include volumes somewhere within this range unless there were clinical indications to use less or more material. The standard protocol in our clinic has been to use 5 and 10 ml of each texture and then allow the patient to drink freely from a cup whenever feasible.

In addition to varying volume, consistency or **viscosity** is varied across swallows. Although variation has been reported across centers and in published reports, general categories of textures include thin liquid, thickened liquid, paste or pudding, and masticated material. The actual thickness or viscosity of a liquid varies across commercial products. A recently developed product line has attempted to standardize the viscosity of barium sulfate liquids into thin, nectar, and honey. A paste material also is available in this product line. One benefit of these standardized barium products is consistency and reproducibility of repeated examinations, both within and across patients. In short, standardized materials reduce variability across examinations that might result from use of different materials.

Sequencing the Events in the Fluoroscopic Study. Initially, the patient is seated and viewed from the lateral perspective. The first tasks often are simple speech or phonation activities to facilitate an impression of movement of structures in the swallowing mechanism (lips, tongue, velum, pharyngeal wall). Subsequently, the initial barium bolus is provided to the patient. Unless there is significant dryness (xerostomia), weakness, or anatomic deviation within the oral cavity structures, the initial bolus is typically 5 ml of thickened liquid. The next material is 5 ml of thin liquid, followed by 5 ml of paste. This sequence is subsequently repeated with 10-ml volumes. Finally, the patient is given a cup of thin liquid barium to drink freely and a masticated material coated with barium paste (usually a cracker).

Following this sequence of events imaged from the lateral view, the patient is turned and viewed from the anterior perspective. From the anterior view, the patient is asked to sustain phonation or to repeat the same vowel so that movement of the true vocal folds can be visualized. Some clinicians also ask the patient to phonate in a falsetto mode to evaluate medial movement of the lateral pharyngeal walls. Turning the patient's head to each side during swallowing may assist in evaluating each hemipharynx and ipsilateral pharyngoesophageal segment (PES) opening. In large part, the materials used in the anterior view depend on the results of swallows examined in the lateral view. In general, not all materials are repeated with the change in orientation, but a sufficient number of swallows are evaluated to assess symmetry, physiology, and the consequences of impaired movement.

Either before or after evaluation of the swallow from the anterior view, compensatory maneuvers might be introduced so that their impact on any observed impairment in swallow physiology can be evaluated. Common compensatory maneuvers include the chin-tuck position, head turn, supraglottic swallow, and Mendelsohn maneuver. Each of these is described in Chapter 10. The impact of these maneuvers can be evaluated in terms of improved swallow safety (less aspiration or penetration) or efficiency (better timing or less residue).

Finally, the esophagus is evaluated whenever feasible. If the patient cannot be positioned appropriately or if the risk of aspiration is too great, esophageal inspection is not added to the standard oropharyngeal examination. Typically, a full esophageal study is not completed at the same time as the oropharyngeal

Box 8-5	*Materials and Sequence of Presentation That May Be Included in a Standardized Fluoroscopic Swallowing Examination*

From Lateral View
- Short speech sample and vowel phonation
- 5 ml of thin liquid barium
- 5 ml of thick liquid barium
- 5 ml of barium paste (pudding)
- 10 ml of thin liquid barium
- 10 ml of thick liquid barium
- 10 ml of barium paste (pudding)
- Thin liquid taken freely from cup or through straw
- Masticated material (cracker coated with barium paste)
- Repeat thin liquid if residue from cracker

From Anterior View (actual material depends on results of lateral view)
- Repeated vowel phonation and falsetto
- Swallow with head forward and turned

Compensatory Maneuvers
- May be introduced at any time in the examination as clinically indicated

Esophageal Evaluation
- Cursory examination for overt obstruction or dysmotility

study. However, a cursory examination of the esophagus may be completed to rule out overt blockages or poor passage of material through the esophagus into the stomach. If the clinical presentation indicates potential for a significant esophageal-based dysphagia and the oropharyngeal examination does not identify any overt difficulties, a more thorough esophagram should be completed.

Clinicians have to decide on how much of the standard protocol to complete for any given patient. Continuing to provide material to a patient who is aspirating a significant amount of each attempted bolus is unwise and contraindicated. Likewise, if a patient becomes excessively fatigued or otherwise unresponsive, a study should not be continued. Blindly following a standard protocol without consideration for the individual needs of the patient is poor practice. Box 8-5 lists the materials and sequence of presentation that may be included in a standardized fluoroscopic swallowing examination.

What to Look for. The short list of what to look for is anatomy and physiology underlying swallowing activity. Initially, anatomic detail and any deviations from normal are to be noted. This includes assessment of the oral cavity structures, velopharynx, pharynx, larynx, PES, and cervical esophagus, as well as the structure of the cervical spine. Depending on the clinical presentation of the patient, anatomy may be viewed from both lateral and anterior perspectives before any physiologic or swallowing assessment is initiated. The lateral view provides the best inspection of the movement within the swallowing mechanism. Box 8-6 summarizes some of the more salient observations that might be obtained from both lateral and anterior views of the fluoroscopic study. Once anatomy of the swallowing mechanism has been reviewed, basic

---

Box 8-6	*Observations That May Be Obtained from the Videofluoroscopic Swallowing Examination*

Anatomy
- All structures

Nonswallow Movement (speech or vowel phonation)
- Lips
- Tongue
- Mandible
- Velum
- Larynx (vocal fold movement from anterior view)
- Pharyngeal walls (falsetto)

Swallow Movement (vary depending on bolus size and consistency)
- Oral containment of liquids anterior and posterior
- Mastication of semisolids and solids
- Oral transit of material into hypopharynx
- Oronasal separation
- Hyoid movement
- Laryngeal elevation and closure
- Pharyngeal contraction
- Pharyngoesophageal segment opening

Consequences of Impaired Swallow Physiology
- Spillage (anterior or posterior)
- Residue
- Misdirection of bolus and airway compromise

Impact of Compensatory Maneuvers (vary depending on impairments)
- Postural adjustment
- Head position changes
- Swallow timing changes (e.g., Mendelsohn maneuver)
- Breath-hold maneuvers
- Bolus changes

---

movement patterns of structures within the swallowing mechanism should be evaluated without swallowing attempts. This practice is useful in understanding any physiologic deficits within the mechanism that may contribute to swallowing problems. Typically, this component of the examination is brief and involves short speech samples or vowel phonation. During these activities, the clinician looks for appropriate movement of the lips, tongue, jaw, velum, larynx, and pharyngeal walls. Movement of the pharyngeal walls can best be evaluated by having the patient produce a falsetto phonation while the clinician views the patient from the anterior perspective. The lateral pharyngeal walls typically move toward the pharyngeal midline with this maneuver.

Following assessment of anatomy and basic movement capabilities of the swallowing mechanism, the clinician advances to direct inspection of swallowing activity. Often, the patient is asked to hold a bolus in the mouth before attempting to swallow. This affords the opportunity to evaluate lip seal anteriorly and linguovelar seal posteriorly. Impairment in these functions results in anterior spillage of the bolus or posterior spillage potentially into an open airway. If a solid bolus is used, clinicians should observe the patient masticate the food material, form a cohesive bolus, and propel this material into the oropharynx. A larger masticated bolus may be swallowed in piecemeal fashion. In this pattern, the patient may deliver small amounts of masticated food into the pharynx while retaining the remaining food in the mouth for further preparation. Whether a liquid or solid bolus is used, the timing and efficiency of oral transit of the bolus should be documented. Poor temporal coordination of the oral component of swallowing might lead to entrance of material into an airway that has not yet closed. Alternatively, a prolonged oral component of swallowing may relate to prolonged mealtimes and thus reduced oral intake and nutritional risk for a patient. Reduced efficiency of oral transport might contribute to residue in and around the oral cavity following the swallowing attempt. This might result from poor motor coordination or from anatomic deficits. Deficits in oronasal separation, whether from anatomic changes or from physiologic deficits in velar movement patterns, can result in entrance of food or liquid into the nasal cavity. This finding is commonly called *nasopharyngeal reflux*. The hyoid bone and larynx typically move as a functional unit during swallowing attempts. Although extensive variation has been described in hyolaryngeal movement, most investigators and clinicians agree that the basic movement is upward and forward (elevation followed by anterior movement of both structures). Although this might sound like a simple activity, appropriate movement of the hyolaryngeal complex involves adequate function of the tongue base and the muscles in the pharyngeal wall. Collectively, these events lead to opening of the PES. In addition, movement of the hyolaryngeal complex is responsible for movement of the epiglottis during swallowing. This latter structure is positioned between the tongue base–hyoid bone and the larynx. As the larynx elevates and the tongue base moves posteriorly and inferiorly, the epiglottis retroflexes to assist in protecting the airway. Deficits in this movement often contribute to postswallow residue in the valleculae anterior to the epiglottis. In addition to elevating within the pharynx, the larynx also closes during the swallowing attempt to protect the airway from entrance of unwanted materials. On the lateral fluoroscopic view, this may be seen as a forward tilting of the arytenoid cartilages approximating the petiole of the epiglottis. As the larynx elevates, the pharynx contracts and, along with tongue-base retropulsion, facilitates passage of the bolus through the hypopharynx into the PES. The PES opens behind the larynx and permits passage of the bolus into the cervical esophagus. Deficits in pharyngeal contraction or PES opening typically result in postswallow residue along the pharyngeal walls and in the piriform sinuses.

If swallow physiology is impaired, clinicians should document the functional consequences of that impairment. Several consequences of impaired swallowing physiology were mentioned previously. Thorough descriptions of postswallow residue and airway compromise in the form of material entering the laryngeal vestibule or aspirated below the true vocal folds should be incorporated into the documentation. These descriptions should include not only the reason for the residue or aspiration, but also the timing of each event and the patient's reaction (or lack thereof) to residue or aspirated material. Finally, the impact of compensatory maneuvers should be investigated and documented. Impact of these maneuvers should be considered not only in terms of changes in observed swallow physiology (e.g., faster swallow, more movement), but also in terms of the functional consequences of these maneuvers (e.g., less residue, improved airway protection).

Strengths and Weaknesses of the Fluoroscopic Swallowing Examination

The videofluoroscopic swallowing examination is considered the "gold standard" in the clinical assessment of dysphagia. This examination has many strengths that merit this designation. It is a dynamic study that, when captured on videotape, provides a thorough evaluation of the biomechanics of oropharyngeal swallowing with unlimited review capability. In addition, it provides a comprehensive perspective on swallowing from the lips through the esophagus. Finally, within the hospital setting it is typically readily accessible for both patient and clinician.

Despite these strengths of the fluoroscopic swallowing examination, weaknesses and questions remain. The use of radiation may be of concern in some instances, especially when multiple, repeated studies are conducted. However, the amount of x-ray in a single examination is quite small. The fluoroscopic examination also is not the best examination to evaluate pooled secretions, because secretions are not visualized with this procedure. Others concerns or areas of question regarding the fluoroscopic swallowing examination might include the following: It documents aspiration but not the effects of aspiration; it may be hard to appreciate airway closure mechanisms; it may not always be accessible outside of the hospital setting; it examines swallow function only for a short time and in an abnormal environment, and thus may not reflect functional eating abilities; transport to the radiology department may be a problem; interpretation may not be reliable among clinicians; and still more issues must be addressed from one patient to the next. This list is not meant to cast aspersions on the videofluoroscopic swallowing examination. Rather, this list should serve as a group of caveats that clinicians may consider when conducting and interpreting this instrumental study.

ENDOSCOPIC SWALLOWING EXAMINATION

Differences Between the Endoscopic Swallowing Examination and the Fluoroscopic Swallowing Examination

Like the fluoroscopic swallowing examination, the endoscopic procedure has been known by a variety of names. Videoendoscopic evaluation of dysphagia (VEED), fiberoptic endoscopic evaluation of dysphagia (FEED), and fiberoptic endoscopic evaluation of swallowing (FEES) have all been used to describe similar procedures. Recently, a position paper endorsed by the ASHA recommended use of the term *FEES* as the generic identifier of this procedure, with the exception of a specific procedure to assess upper airway sensitivity (fiberoptic endoscopic evaluation of swallowing with sensory testing [FEESST]). In keeping with the discussion of the fluoroscopic examination, this chapter continues to use the generic descriptive term *endoscopic swallowing examination*.

The endoscopic swallowing examination is newer than the fluoroscopic examination in the clinical arena of dysphagia, and therefore is used by fewer

| Box 8-7 | *Similarities and Differences Between the Fluoroscopic and Endoscopic Swallow Studies* |

Similarities	**Differences**
• Purpose	• Technique
• Materials	• Image perspective
• Process of evaluation	• Portability
	• Repeatability
	• Duration of examination
	• Sensory assessment

professionals. Nevertheless, this instrumental examination is growing in popularity and application and shares both similarities and differences with the fluoroscopic study. Box 8-7 summarizes some of the more salient similarities and differences between these two instrumental procedures for the assessment of swallowing function.

Similarities. Both procedures have a similar purpose in the assessment of swallowing. Each is intended to provide an objective assessment of the anatomy and physiology of the upper aerodigestive mechanisms used in swallowing. Although each procedure has advantages or disadvantages over the other, both are intended for a similar purpose. Materials used in both examinations vary in amount and texture. The fluoroscopic study uses barium sulfate as a visible contrast agent, whereas the endoscopic study uses liquids and foods of natural or added color to be visible. Thus both studies use a range of liquid and solid foods that are designed to be easily visualized by the respective examinations. Finally, both studies use a similar assessment process. Both procedures allow the clinician to evaluate anatomy and physiology of the upper swallow mechanism, swallow function, and the impact of compensatory maneuvers.

Differences. Differences between the procedures include obvious technique differences. Beyond technique differences, the resulting images from the respective procedures differ. Fluoroscopy is considered to provide the more comprehensive perspective including structures from the lips to the stomach. Endoscopy has imaging capability focused on the pharynx from the nasopharynx to the hypopharynx. Oral cavity and esophageal structure and function are not part of the typical endoscopic swallowing examination. In addition, whereas the endoscopic image is lost at the peak of the swallow or in those instances where material covers the end of the endoscope, the fluoroscopic image suffers no similar limitations. Figure 8-3 compares a clear endoscopic image, an image impaired by secretions on the endoscope, and a "white-out" image that occurs at the swallowing peak. Despite the potential for image degradation during the endoscopic examination, this procedure is superior to fluoroscopy in the evaluation of both anatomy and pooled secretion within the swallowing mechanism. Another advantage of the endoscopic procedure is the potential for portability. Endoscopic systems are available that can be transported with relative ease to the patient in various locations, thus increasing access to this examination. Because endoscopy does not involve

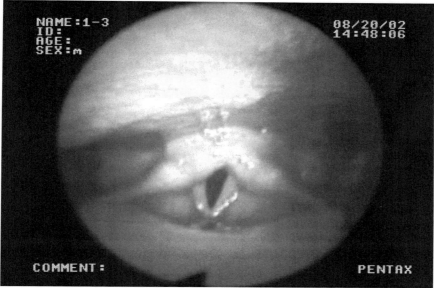

A

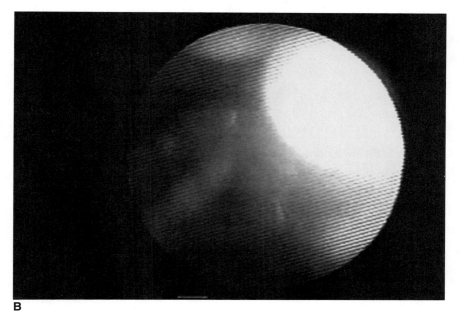

B

FIGURE 8-3 A clear endoscopic image of the pharynx (**A**), an image obscured by secretions on the endoscope (**B**), and an example of "white out" (**C**).

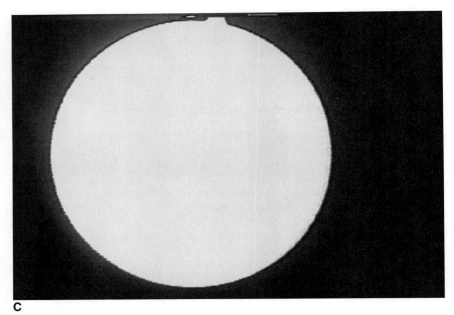

C

FIGURE 8-3 Cont'd.
For legend see previous page.

x-ray radiation, repeated examinations are not viewed with as much concern as are repeated fluoroscopic examinations. In addition, because no x-ray is used, individual endoscopic examinations can be somewhat longer than fluoroscopic examination. Finally, with the endoscopic procedure, sensory functions may be tested, albeit crudely, by touching the mucosa and asking the patient to acknowledge the tactile stimulus.

Procedures for the Endoscopic Swallowing Examination

The endoscopic swallowing examination includes five components: (1) assessment of pharyngeal anatomy (including laryngeal structures), (2) evaluation of movement and sensation of pharyngeal structures, (3) assessment of secretions, (4) direct evaluation of swallowing function with liquid and solid material, and (5) evaluation of the impact of compensatory maneuvers.

Specialized equipment is required for the endoscopic swallowing examination. The minimal requirements for an adequate endoscopic system for evaluation of swallowing function include a fiberoptic endoscope, a light source, a camera, and a video recording system. These basic elements are depicted in Figure 8-4.

The first step in the endoscopic swallowing examination should be patient instruction. This is especially important for patients undergoing the examination for the first time. The **transnasal** endoscopic procedure is not painful, but it may be uncomfortable for some individuals. Whenever possible, the procedure should be thoroughly explained to the patient.

The next issue is whether to use nasal anesthesia. Historically, both a **vasoconstrictor** and an anesthetic have been sprayed into the nose before the

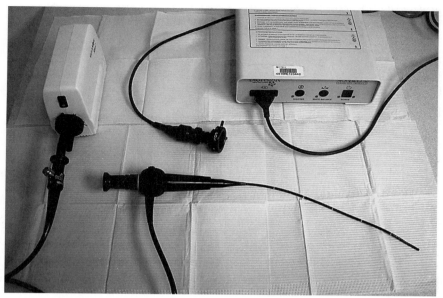

FIGURE 8-4 Basic equipment required for the endoscopic swallowing examination: endoscope, light source, and camera (video recording system not shown).

procedure. However, recent research has provided convincing evidence that neither medication is required for most examinations. If used, these medications should be applied only under direct medical supervision, because all medications have potential side effects.

Initially, the clinician passes the fiberoptic endoscope through one nasal passage, taking care to stay in the **inferior nasal meatus** and away from the nasal septum. Once in the nasal **choana**, the scope may be positioned to view the velopharynx. (*Note:* Experienced endoscopists realize that to get the optimal view of the velopharynx, the scope should be placed in the middle nasal meatus. However, this can contribute to increased discomfort for the patient.) Function of the velopharyngeal mechanism can be examined by asking the patient to hum, to produce vowels and consonants, and to verbalize short sentences. Initially, a dry (saliva only) swallow is completed to assess velar movement during swallowing. If nasopharyngeal reflux is suspected, this can be evaluated initially by looking for saliva passing through the velopharyngeal port during the dry swallow. It is preferable not to give the patient material to swallow at this point, but to wait until the airway is clearly visualized.

Following inspection of the velopharyngeal mechanism, the scope is advanced into the oropharynx, with the tip positioned below the uvula and above the epiglottis. From this position, the pharynx should be well visualized, including laryngeal structures. Figure 8-5 presents the normal anatomic views from this position of the abducted and adducted larynx. The reader should refer to the video accompanying this text for anatomic details

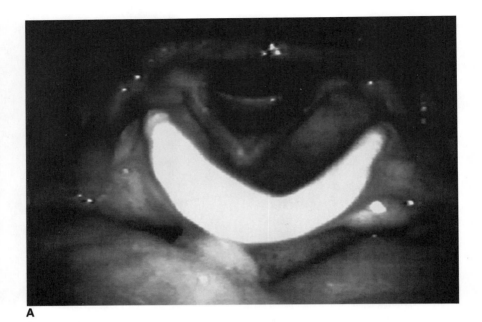

A

B

FIGURE 8-5 Normal endoscopic view of abducted **(A)** and adducted **(B)** larynx.

(Crary and Groher, *Video Introduction to Adult Swallowing Disorders,* Butterworth-Heinemann). Assessment techniques for pharyngeal activities include asking the patient to produce falsetto phonation, perform a Valsalva maneuver, and swallow various materials. Falsetto phonation facilitates medial movement of the lateral pharyngeal walls; this activity is a good method to identify hemipharyngeal weakness. The pharyngeal wall demonstrating little or no movement is likely to be paretic. The Valsalva maneuver is a method used to expand the pharynx. This view may be helpful in identifying subtle anatomic deviations or as an indication of weakness on one side of the pharynx.

Assessment of laryngeal function includes activities for both adduction and abduction and for diadochokinesis, breath-hold, and cough and clear actions. Simple phonation is adequate for laryngeal adduction. The vowel "ee" is used most often because it elongates the larynx and enhances the endoscopic view. Abduction may be evaluated by forced inhalation or sniffing. Laryngeal diadochokinesis may be assessed by alternating phonation and sniffing or by repeated productions of the syllable "see" or "he." Breath-hold maneuvers should include both a simple breath-hold ("hold your breath") and a forced breath-hold ("hold your breath and bear down"). It is well recognized that many adults do not completely close the larynx with a simple breath-hold. Laryngeal closure is typically achieved with forced breath-hold, barring significant anatomic or physiologic deficit. In instances in which a breath-hold maneuver may be incorporated into a therapy program, it is important to know whether a simple breath-hold will achieve glottal closure or whether a forced breath-hold is indicated. Finally, it is important to ascertain the patient's ability to execute a voluntary cough and decide whether that cough is sufficient to clear any pooled secretions or mucus from the vocal folds and/or laryngeal vestibule.

Attempted swallows should be completed with a range of materials that are clearly visible under endoscopic inspection. The selection and sequential presentation of materials to be swallowed follows concepts similar to the selection and sequential presentation of materials used during the fluoroscopic examination. During each swallow, a period of "white out" occurs at the point of maximal pharyngeal contraction. Following the swallow, the pharynx and larynx are again visible, and assessment of airway compromise via penetration and/or aspiration and patterns of residue may be performed. Again, although the view is different, the concepts of what to look for in the endoscopic examination are similar to those for the fluoroscopic examination. If impaired swallow physiology is identified, compensatory maneuvers may be implemented under endoscopic inspection to evaluate their impact on both the impaired physiology and the consequences of that impairment.

Strengths and Weakness of the Endoscopic Swallowing Examination

Like the fluoroscopic swallowing examination, the endoscopic procedure is a dynamic study that, when captured on videotape, provides an objective examination of pharyngeal swallowing function with review capability. It provides a superior inspection of pharyngeal anatomy, sensation, laryngeal closure patterns, and secretions compared with fluoroscopy. Accessibility is deemed a strength of the endoscopic procedure secondary to portability, and repeated assessments pose no concern of x-ray exposure. Some clinicians and researchers have used this technique in repeated applications as a biofeed-back tool, specifically to teach patients airway protection strategies. Finally, swallowing examinations with this procedure can conceivably be longer than those performed with the fluoroscopic procedure, because no radiation is involved.

Perhaps the biggest limitation of the endoscopic swallowing examination is the relatively limited scope of view. Unlike the fluoroscopic study, this procedure does not provide imaging of the oral cavity or the esophagus. The focus of the image and thus evaluation is clearly on pharyngeal aspects of swallowing. The issue of "white out" during the swallowing peak has been raised as a potential limitation of this procedure; however, in practice, this brief period of image loss rarely impacts the outcome of the evaluation, and in some instances, the absence of this normal finding implicates a weakened pharyngeal swallow. Safety issues have been raised regarding this procedure, with potential complications including nosebleed, **laryngospasm, vasovagal response**, and allergic reaction to medications when used. However, published reports of relatively large numbers of patients receiving this procedure have documented that it is a safe procedure with few complications. Additional research has demonstrated that neither anesthetics nor vasoconstrictors are necessary to complete this procedure. However, patient safety must be a primary concern in any clinical setting. Patients who may be combative, who demonstrate movement disorders that might preclude completion of a safe examination, or who have bleeding disorders might increase any risk factor associated with this procedure.

One final limitation of the endoscopic swallowing examination merits consideration. Before engaging in either the application or the interpretation of endoscopic swallowing examinations, clinicians must avail themselves of an appropriate degree of supervised training. (Of course, this same concern should be addressed for the fluoroscopic study.) Published guidelines are available from the ASHA that detail the knowledge and skills required to undertake this procedure and that suggest mechanisms to obtain appropriate training.

DIRECT COMPARISONS BETWEEN THE FLUOROSCOPIC AND ENDOSCOPIC SWALLOWING EXAMINATIONS

Several investigations have undertaken direct comparisons between the fluoroscopic and endoscopic swallowing examinations. Some of these comparisons have been practical suggestions for application based on clinical experience, whereas others have been more rigorous comparisons of specific findings on the respective procedures in common groups of patients with dysphagia. As mentioned previously, one advantage of the fluoroscopic procedure is a more comprehensive evaluation of swallowing from lips to stomach. Based on this advantage, the fluoroscopic procedure has been advocated as the preferred procedure for initial swallowing assessments and for instrumental assessment of dysphagia symptoms focused on the esophagus. Conversely, the endoscopic procedure provides a superior inspection of anatomy and secretions. Based on this advantage, the endoscopic procedure has been advocated

Table 8-1	Relative Clinical Advantages and Uses of the Fluoroscopic and Endoscopic Swallowing Examinations		
APPLICATION		**ADVANTAGE FLUOROSCOPY**	**ADVANTAGE ENDOSCOPY**
Initial evaluation		X	
Esophageal dysphagia		X	
Paresis/paralysis (cranial nerve)			X
Anatomic deviations			X
Secretion evaluation			X
Patient who cannot be transported			X
Repeated use			X
Biofeedback			X

in cases involving paralysis secondary to cranial neuropathies or involving postsurgical or traumatic anatomic changes, as well as for any dysphagia in which the management and/or aspiration of secretions is problematic. Finally, because of the portability advantage of the endoscopic procedure and the absence of radiation exposure, it has been advocated for patients who are not able to be transported (i.e., bedfast patients), for situations requiring repeated swallowing examinations, and for use as a biofeedback application in treatment. These advocated clinical preferences are summarized in Table 8-1.

Studies comparing specific findings between these two instrumental procedures have consistently identified a high degree of agreement. Table 8-2 summarizes the results of three studies comparing various swallowing deficits. Findings of residue or airway compromise reveal agreement averaging from 80% to 90% between these two procedures. Other studies comparing these instrumental examinations also have reported strong agreement on a number of dysphagia characteristics. Given the high agreement reported between these procedures and the specific advantages attributed to each, it is apparent that depending on the requirements of the clinical situation, one procedure might be indicated over the other or that the two procedures might be used in a complementary fashion during the same dysphagia evaluation.

Table 8-2	Results of Three Studies Comparing Specific Findings of the Fluoroscopic and Endoscopic Swallowing Examinations*		
FINDING	**STUDY #1**	**STUDY #2**	**STUDY #3**
Pharyngeal residue	80%	89%	92%
Aspiration	90%	86%	Before: 100% During: 84% After: 96%
Laryngeal penetration	85%	86%	Did not test
Premature spillage (posterior)	66%	61%	Did not test

*Numbers reflect percentage agreement between the two instrumental examinations.

TAKE HOME NOTES

- Instrumental studies of swallowing provide objective imaging of the anatomy and physiology of the swallowing mechanism and swallowing biomechanics across varying bolus and patient conditions.
- Instrumental studies of swallowing should be strongly considered whenever a thorough clinical evaluation is insufficient to answer the pertinent clinical questions for a given patient. This may include delineation of dysphagia parameters, clarification of airway protection issues, the impact of compensatory maneuvers, and/or monitoring change over time. These examinations may also provide information that is useful in understanding medical conditions that underlie dysphagia.
- Commonalities exist between procedures for the fluoroscopic and endoscopic swallowing examinations. Both provide dynamic imaging of the swallowing mechanism and performance, use multiple bolus volumes and textures, and have the potential to evaluate the impact of compensatory maneuvers on swallowing safety and efficiency. In addition, each may be modified to address individual needs of specific patient groups or dysphagia characteristics.
- Both instrumental swallowing examinations have strengths and weaknesses that might impact when they are most useful. The fluoroscopic study offers the more comprehensive perspective of the swallowing mechanism, whereas the endoscopic study offers the superior view of anatomy and secretions. Certain weaknesses are common to both procedures. They may document the presence of aspiration but do not address the consequences of aspiration. They evaluate swallowing performance in abnormal environments using procedures that do not resemble functional eating activities. Despite these potential criticisms, these examinations do have a critical role in the assessment of swallowing performance.
- Published reports indicate strong agreement between the fluoroscopic and endoscopic swallowing examinations, specifically in the identification of individual dysphagia characteristics such as postswallow residue and aspiration. Agreement in the identification of specific clinical findings along with consideration of the relative strengths and weaknesses of each procedure helps with the appropriate application of either or both procedures.

CASE EXAMPLES

CASE 1

An 85-year-old woman is seen in the outpatient dysphagia clinic. She currently resides in a long-term care facility. Facility staff is concerned because the patient is declining food and is beginning to lose weight. In addition, she has been reported to cough during mealtimes. Her adult son accompanied her to the evaluation and served as the primary informant. He visits his mother at least twice each week and has observed mealtimes and participated in feeding her. The patient is unable to self-feed secondary to severe arthritis in her hands. She has a moderate dementia but is able to communicate her preferences and dislikes with simple responses. She is on a total oral diet of pureed foods and thickened liquids. She indicates that she does not like this diet and that the food has no taste. On occasion, the family has brought regular food to her and observed her eat without difficulty. Clinical examination revealed neither gross abnormality in cranial nerve function nor any anatomic deviations in the oral structures. Her voice was deemed appropriate for her age and medical condition. Volitional cough was intact. The patient was provided a range of material to swallow based on the report of her daily oral intake. Initially, thickened liquids were presented on a spoon. The patient was able to swallow these without difficulty and without postswallow voice change. Larger amounts of thickened liquid were provided in a cup. Again, no difficulties were detected. Subsequently, thin liquid (fruit juice) was provided, first by spoon, then by cup, then by straw. A single cough was observed following cup drinking. No difficulties were observed during straw drinking. Pudding was presented in spoon-size attempts. Lingual mastication was evident and no difficulties were observed. Subsequently, a cracker was presented. Mastication was obvious, but oral residue was observed following swallow attempts. Thin liquid was presented through a straw to clear the oral residue. No overt signs of aspiration were noted and her voice was clear after drinking. Oral residue was cleared with straw drinking.

Interpretation This patient did not require any instrumental examination for swallowing function. Clinical examination with swallowing evaluation was sufficient in addressing the concerns regarding her refusal of food and the occasional coughing during meals. Recommendations for this patient included upgrading her diet to soft mechanical or further, depending on preference and tolerance, and allowing her to drink thin liquids. An occupational therapy consult was generated to fashion a cup-holding device that would allow the patient to drink thin liquids (specifically water) through a straw at her discretion. Follow-up with this patient indicated that the recommendations were implemented, food and liquid intake increased, and no dysphagia-related complications were encountered.

CASE 2

A 64-year-old man comes to the dysphagia clinic following radiation therapy for a tonsillar fossa carcinoma. The patient complained of dry mouth (xerostomia), which made it difficult to swallow dry, solid foods and moderate pain in his throat, which was worse with any swallow. He had no overt cranial nerve deficits, but his voice was mildly hoarse (he reported that this was a result of the radiation therapy). He reported that he consistently coughed to clear thickened secretions from his throat.

Interpretation The patient showed several indications for completion of an endoscopic swallowing examination. He was post–radiation therapy, which can contribute to xerostomia, mucositis, anatomic changes, and even, physiologic changes in pharyngeal structures used in swallowing. He demonstrated voice changes, meriting inspection of the laryngeal valve, and he complained of pooling of thickened secretions. Endoscopic swallowing examination revealed thickened secretions bilaterally in the piriform sinuses and, to a lesser degree, within the laryngeal vestibule. The vocal folds were mobile but **edematous** and **erythematous,** suggesting irritation, and the left vocal fold was slightly bowed, creating a small glottal gap during phonation. Swallowing attempts of various consistencies revealed no difficulties with thin or thick liquids but mild postswallow residue in the hypopharynx for pudding and masticated materials. This residue was completely cleared with subsequent swallows of thin liquid. Based on the results of this examination, no fluoroscopic study was completed. Recommendations were to continue total oral feeding, to moisten the mouth before ingesting pudding or solid materials, to use liquids to clear residue from more-solid foods, and to consult his oncologist for treatment of mucositis.

CASE 3
A 76-year-old man complains of swallowing difficulty following hemispheric stroke. His primary complaint is that food sticks, and he localizes the problem to the base of the neck just above the sternum. He complains of having excess saliva that causes him to cough. His cough is weak and his voice is dysphonic and breathy.

Interpretation This patient had dysphagia complaints that required both endoscopic and fluoroscopic swallowing examinations. Difficulty managing secretions, weak cough, and voice changes are indications for completing an endoscopic examination of pharyngeal and laryngeal functions. Complaints of food sticking at the level of the neck base indicate the need to complete a fluoroscopic examination. Endoscopic examination revealed a left vocal fold paresis with incomplete glottal closure and pooled "foamy" secretions throughout the hypopharynx and in the laryngeal vestibule. Falsetto maneuver revealed a paretic left hemipharynx. Swallow attempts revealed postswallow residue in the left piriform sinus that increased as the viscosity of the swallowed material increased. Fluoroscopic swallowing examination confirmed a left hemipharyngeal paresis and incomplete opening of the PES, with less opening on the left side. Recommendations initially focused on referral to an otolaryngologist for consideration of vocal fold medialization and procedures to improve PES opening.

CHAPTER TERMS

choana a funnel-shaped opening; in this case, meaning the space in the posterior nasal cavity behind the nasal septum

contrast agent in radiology, a foreign substance used to provide a different density so that tissue can be better visualized; positive-contrast agents appear black on radiograph to better delineate the adjacent tissue and air spaces, which are lighter

edematous swollen

erythematous redness

inferior nasal meatus the inferior passage from the nasal entrance to the choana, below the inferior turbinate

laryngospasm spasm of the laryngeal muscles, which may contribute to reduced ability to breathe

radiopaque impenerable to x-rays or other forms of radiation; opposite of radiolucent or radioparent

transnasal literally meaning "across the nose"; in this case, meaning passing an endoscope through the nose

vasoconstrictor a substance that causes constriction of blood vessels; in this context, a vasoconstrictor is used to "shrink" nasal tissues, resulting in a larger passage through which to pass an endoscope

vasovagal response sudden fainting from stimulation to the vagus nerve, accompanied by pallor, sweating, hyperventilation, and bradycardia
viscosity resistance of a fluid; in simple terms, the thickness of a fluid

SUGGESTED READINGS

American Speech-Language-Hearing Association (ASHA): *Clinical indicators for instrumental assessment of dysphagia (guidelines): ASHA desk reference,* Rockville, Md, 2000, ASHA.

American Speech-Language-Hearing Association (ASHA): *Knowledge and skills for speech-language pathologists performing endoscopic assessment of swallowing function,* ASHA Supplement 22, 2002. Available at www.professional.asha.org.

Aviv JE: Prospective, randomized outcome study of endoscopy versus modified barium swallow in patients with dysphagia, *Laryngoscope* 110:563, 2000.

Aviv JE et al: Air pulse quantification of supraglottic and pharyngeal sensation: a new technique, *Ann Otol Rhinol Laryngol* 102:777, 1993.

Aviv JE et al: The safety of flexible endoscopic evaluation of swallowing with sensory testing (FEESST): an analysis of 500 consecutive evaluations, *Dysphagia* 15:39, 2000.

Bastian R: Videoendoscopic evaluation of patients with dysphagia: an adjunct to the modified barium swallow, *Otolaryngol Head Neck Surg* 3:339, 1991.

Bastian R: The videoendoscopic swallowing study: an alternative and partner to the videofluoroscopic swallowing study, *Dysphagia* 8:359, 1993.

Crary MA, Baron J: Endoscopic and fluoroscopic evaluations of swallowing: comparison of observed and inferred findings, *Dysphagia* 2:108, 1997.

Kendall KA, Leonard RJ, McKenzie SW: Accommodation to changes in bolus viscosity in normal deglutition: a videofluoroscopic study, *Ann Otol Rhinol Laryngol* 110:1059, 2001.

Kendall KA et al: Timing of events in normal swallowing: a videofluoroscopic study, *Dysphagia* 15:74, 2000.

Kidder TM, Langmore SE, Martin BJ: Indications and techniques of endoscopy in evaluation of cervical dysphagia: comparison with radiographic techniques, *Dysphagia* 9:256, 1994.

Kuhlemeier KV, Yates P, Palmer JB: Intra- and interrater variation in the evaluation of videofluorographic swallowing studies, *Dysphagia* 13:142, 1998.

Langmore SE: *Endoscopic evaluation and treatment of swallowing disorders,* New York, 2000, Thieme.

Langmore SE, Schatz K, Olson N: Endoscopic and videofluoroscopic evaluations of swallowing and aspiration, *Ann Otol Rhinol Laryngol* 100:678, 1991.

Leonard RJ et al: Structural displacements in normal swallowing: a videofluoroscopic study, *Dysphagia* 15:146, 2000.

Logemann JA: *Manual for the videofluorographic study of swallowing,* Boston, 1986, Little, Brown and Company.

Logemann JA et al: Effectiveness of four hours of education in interpretation of radiographic studies, *Dysphagia* 15:180, 2000.

Madden C et al: Comparison between videofluoroscopy and milk-swallow endoscopy in the assessment of swallowing function, *Clin Otolaryngol* 25:504, 2000.

Martin BJ et al: Normal laryngeal valving patterns during three breath-holding maneuvers: a pilot investigation, *Dysphagia* 8:11, 1993.

Mendelsohn MS, Martin R: Airway protection during breath holding, *Ann Otol Rhinol Laryngol* 102:941, 1993.

Murray J: *Manual of dysphagia assessment in adults,* San Diego, 1999, Singular Publishing Group.

Ott DJ: Observer variation in evaluation of videofluoroscopic swallowing studies: a continuing problem, *Dysphagia* 13:148, 1998.

Robbins J et al: Differentiation of normal and abnormal airway protection during swallowing using the penetration-aspiration scale, *Dysphagia* 14:228, 1999.

Schroter-Morasch H et al: Values and limitations of pharyngolaryngoscopy (transnasal, transoral) in patients with dysphagia, *Folia Phoniatr Logop* 51:172, 1999.

Singh V, Brockbank MJ, Todd GB: Flexible transnasal endoscopy: is local anaesthetic necessary? *J Laryngol Otol* 111:616, 1997.

Spinelli KS, Easterling CS, Shaker R: Radiographic evaluation of complex dysphagic patients: comparison with videoendoscopic technique, *Curr Gastroenterol Rep* 4:187, 2002.

Wilcox F, Liss JM, Siegel GM: Interjudge agreement in videofluoroscopic studies of swallowing, *J Speech Hear Res* 39:144, 1996.

Wooi M, Scott A, Perry A: Teaching speech pathology students the interpretation of videofluoroscopic swallowing studies, *Dysphagia* 16:32, 2001.

Wu CH et al: Evaluation of swallowing safety with fiberoptic endoscope: comparison with videofluoroscopic technique, *Laryngoscope* 107:396, 1997.

CHAPTER 9

Treatment Considerations, Options, and Decisions

FOCUS QUESTIONS

1 What are two primary treatment considerations that apply to most dysphagia cases? Discuss various implications of these considerations.

2 What are some possible objectives of dysphagia therapy? Discuss general factors that influence therapy decisions.

3 What are some practical considerations that may apply in choosing specific therapy techniques?

4 What are the major categories of treatment for dysphagia? Give examples of specific techniques within each category.

5 Which aspects of the evaluation process might dysphagia clinicians use to obtain information related to specific aspects of treatment? Discuss how evaluation information may impact treatment planning.

6 What simple steps may be followed to formulate meaningful clinical questions addressing choice of therapy technique?

7 What specific steps may be followed in developing a treatment plan for an individual patient with dysphagia?

GENERAL CONSIDERATIONS FOR DYSPHAGIA TREATMENT

Treatment planning for the dysphagic patient requires many considerations drawn from an extensive information base. Clinicians must not only be aware of multiple factors that may impact treatment decisions, but they also must be aware of where they can obtain information needed to make those decisions. In general, both the patient and the choice of treatment technique bring unique questions to the clinical decision-making task.

A pair of common considerations inherent to all aspects of dysphagia is airway protection and nutrition and hydration. Clinicians often face the important question, *"Can the patient safely resume or increase adequate oral intake?"* Dissecting this question reveals critical considerations in dysphagia treatment. The primary concerns for dysphagia patients may be found in the words *safe* and *adequate*. Safety is often expressed in terms of airway protection. Patients who aspirate most of any given bolus of food or liquid are not considered safe in reference to the risk of aspiration and subsequent respiratory infection or, possibly, the risk of airway obstruction from more solid foods. The reference to *adequate* refers to the individual's ability to ingest sufficient food or liquid by mouth to maintain (or increase, if required in the situation) nutrition and hydration. A patient who engages in total oral feeding only to ingest inadequate volumes of food or liquid is a patient who is at risk for future health problems. When patients are using only nonoral feeding routes, the focus of treatment should be on the potential to resume oral intake of food and liquid. If the patient is taking a total oral diet, the focus may be on expanding the amount of intake to enhance nutrition, or the focus may be on expanding the variety of the diet to improve social aspects of eating and presumably quality of life. In planning treatment, it is important to have a clear grasp of the patient's present situation and a clear vision of where both clinician and patient want to be in the future and the factors that may help or hinder that direction.

In selecting any therapy, consideration must be given to the objective of that therapy. For example, in medicine one goal of therapy might be to cure a disease. How do clinicians "cure" dysphagia? Does curing dysphagia suggest that clinicians must return nonoral feeding patients to oral feeding? This is not always possible. Do clinicians want to prevent recurrence of a dysphagia-related comorbidity? One potential example might be to diminish or eliminate recurrent chest infections. This certainly provides direction in treatment planning. In some situations, clinicians may focus on limiting functional deterioration or facilitating recovery. To adopt this focus, clinicians must have a clear understanding of the underlying conditions contributing to dysphagia in individual patients. Certainly, clinicians hope that interventions do not contribute to later complications and that they, in fact, contribute to prevention of complications such as chest infections and malnutrition.

Beyond specific goals of treatment, clinicians must consider the nature of the swallowing deficit and the treatment options available to them and the patient (these are not always the same). Box 9-1 summarizes some issues that might be addressed regarding the swallowing deficit. A basic question might revolve around feeding versus swallowing processes: Are there physical or cognitive factors that preclude successful feeding but that do not interfere with swallowing function? Are both of these factors present, and if so, do they interact in a positive or negative manner? Certain dysphagia-causing diseases might demonstrate differences between voluntary or involuntary motor processes. If differences are present, are there swallowing activities that may be used to tap into voluntary versus involuntary motor processes? Stage of deficit is an artificial delineation often used for convenience. Are the swallowing deficits primarily located within the oral, oropharyngeal, pharyngeal, or esophageal component? Clinicians must also remember that not only are these "stages" artificial, but that the swallowing mechanism is interactive, in that events occurring in one anatomic area have the potential to impact performance in another area. A difficult clinical task can be attempting to separate the specific swallowing deficit from any compensatory activities used by individual patients. For example, consider the patient who attempts to

| Box 9-1 | *Treatment Considerations Focusing on the Nature of the Swallowing Deficit* |

- Feeding or swallowing deficits (or both)
- Voluntary or involuntary processes
- Stage of deficit
- Deficit or compensatory activity

swallow but immediately begins to expectorate the bolus and demonstrates a pattern of "mini swallows" interspersed with throat clearing, resulting in only a minute amount of material actually being swallowed. Does this pattern reflect a specific pattern of impaired physiology? Does it reflect the presence of compensations intended to protect the airway, or are there other possibilities? In some cases, this distinction may not be important. However, in others, it may be important to understand what might be changed as a result of therapy versus what might not be changed. This consideration may impact the decision to engage in therapy and, if so, the direction of that therapy.

An additional point worthy of emphasis is that dysphagia treatment is rarely unifocal. Dysphagia is the result of underlying disease or disorder processes. Consequently, patients with dysphagia often receive therapies from medical, surgical, and/or behavioral realms. Clinicians who are treating patients with dysphagia should be aware of concomitant treatments, as well as dysphagia treatments in other realms that may either work together or in place of behavioral treatment strategies. Figure 9-1 is a schematic reminder of how these therapy categories may interact. In certain clinical situations, one category may comprise the primary or sole treatment approach. In other situations, two or all three categories may interact to form the most beneficial intervention.

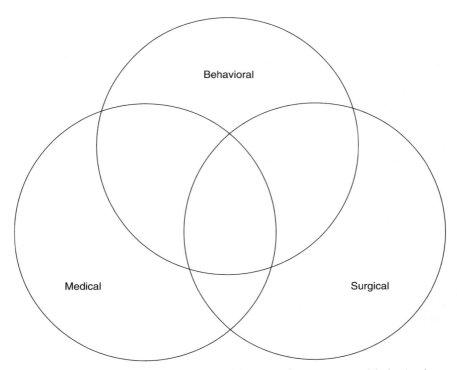

FIGURE 9-1 A schematic representation of potential interactions of behavioral, medical, and surgical treatment options in dysphagia.

TREATMENT CONSIDERATIONS SPECIFIC TO THE PATIENT

Patients bring to any clinical situation a plethora of circumstances, which are typically unique from one person to the next. Box 9-2 offers a list of potential patient-related considerations that may impact dysphagia treatment options and decisions. As stated many times throughout this text, dysphagia is the result of underlying disease processes. The cause of dysphagia should be understood as best as clinically possible, because the underlying disease presents a clinical course that has direct impact on swallowing function and benefits from various intervention strategies over time.

Severity of dysphagia is a more complex concept than might be imagined at first consideration. How is the severity of dysphagia graded? Some clinicians and investigators have used impairment of swallowing physiology based on instrumental examination, whereas others have used more functional measures of amount of food or liquid taken by mouth. Some clinicians may believe that patients who take no food by mouth also have the poorest swallowing physiology. Unfortunately, this is not always the case. Patient status may change over time, and some patients who receive only nonoral feeding may actually have adequate swallowing physiology to ingest some degree of food or liquid by mouth. Thus severity of dysphagia should not be considered a unitary concept, because many factors are involved.

Eating history may provide clinicians with some idea of a patient's motivation and willingness to push himself or herself toward increased oral intake. This interacts directly with certain psychosocial considerations. For example, the patient who reports that he "lives to eat, not eats to live" and who engages in the practice of chewing food that cannot be swallowed just to get the taste may be more compliant with a rigorous therapy plan than the patient who uses only nonoral sources and never attempts any oral intake of food or liquid. In addition, eating history may provide the clinician with cultural biases in food selection (i.e., the patient never ate that food or always ate that food) or limitations in specific food availability associated with the patient's environment. Social aspects of eating should also be considered, in terms of the patient's current situation ("I attempt to eat alone in my room") and his or her aspirations ("I would like to eat in a restaurant"). Finally, for patients who engage in both oral and tube feeding, eating history may explain the timing of one form of feeding relative to the other. This may be important in reaching functional goals in therapy.

Anticipated medical course is an essential factor for the clinician to understand. It may impact not only the consideration of whether to initiate therapy, but also which types of therapy to undertake. In some clinical scenarios, it may

---

Box 9-2	*Treatment Considerations Focusing on Patient Characteristics*

- Etiology (underlying disease or disorder)
- Severity
- Eating history

- Psychosocial factors
- Anticipated medical course
- Caregiver factors

be better to wait and monitor the patient's condition (e.g., stability, endurance). In other situations, aggressive therapy is indicated. Clinicians must keep in mind that therapeutic strategies should change as the patient's underlying condition (and potentially dysphagia) changes.

Caregiver considerations are an extension of patient considerations, especially for patients (at any age) who are unable to perform self-care (including feeding). Whether the caregiver is a nurse, other qualified health care provider, spouse or other family member, or friend, caregiver performance can have a direct impact (positive or negative) on the performance of the dysphagic patient. Mealtimes can become complicated by a caregiver who is uninitiated in proper feeding strategies for the dependent patient. Positioning of the patient, rate and manner of food presentation, and other variables need to be clear to caregivers.

The environment in which the dysphagia patient resides also can impact the nature of dysphagia intervention (see Chapter 1). The needs of the patient in the intensive care unit are different from those of the individual receiving outpatient therapy. In addition, the resources available in different environments differ dramatically. Clinicians working in academic medical centers often experience more available resources than do clinicians working in rural long-term care facilities.

TREATMENT CONSIDERATIONS SPECIFIC TO CHOICE OF APPROACH OR TECHNIQUE

Treatment techniques (including medical, surgical, and behavioral), like individual patients, require specific consideration in planning intervention. As mentioned previously, treatment options change as the patient changes over time. From this perspective, the decision of when to intervene, as well as how to intervene (choice of technique), changes according to the patient's condition. In general, treatment strategies may be considered in reference to the degree of interaction with the patient and/or the intent of treatment. A common approach to patients who are severely debilitated or in the acute phase of an illness is a prophylactic or preventative approach. These approaches often tend to be passive, not requiring substantial activity from the patient. Oral hygiene, passive movements, and perhaps diet changes might be considered passive interventions. Active interventions are those in which the patient is required to engage in direct maneuvers or compensations to change some aspect of swallowing performance. Another dichotomy that may overlap with active versus passive interventions is that of patient-centered versus environment-centered interventions. Patient-centered interventions may be active or passive, but all focus on the patient. Environment-centered interventions are primarily passive, with the focus on changing some aspect of the patient's environment. Dysphagia dining rooms or special mealtimes are examples of environment-centered interventions.

Considering the Choice of Treatments

Box 9-3 presents a list of considerations that apply in choosing any specific treatment technique. Clinicians must consider which treatment options are realistically available to them. In determining whether a treatment option is

Box 9-3	*Considerations in Choosing a Specific Treatment Technique*

• Options	What?
• Clinical indicators	Why?
• Anticipated risks and benefits	Immediate
• Functional outcome	Long term
• Patient empowerment	Compliance

realistically available, the following should be considered: the physical presence of technology required to use a specific technique (e.g., surface electromyography [sEMG] biofeedback), the clinician's knowledge of and skill at performing a specific technique, and the patient's acceptance of the technique. (Does the patient understand the instructions? Is he or she able to perform the technique? Can the patient afford the technique? What are the demands on the patient to adequately perform the technique?)

Clinical indicators address the question, "Why choose this particular technique?" For example, how does the technique under consideration relate to the specifics of the patient's dysphagia complaints or symptoms? Is the technique clinically and biologically plausible? Should the technique be performed in isolation or in combination with other techniques? These considerations are important in selecting any specific technique.

Anticipated risks and benefits to the patient should be considered in reference to the immediate outcome of the technique. Some techniques that appear to be relatively benign may complicate certain comorbidities in some patients. For example, techniques that emphasize a prolonged **apneic pause** during swallowing attempts might be problematic for some patients with significant respiratory diseases. (See Chapter 4 for another example.) Techniques that require significant muscular effort during repeated swallow attempts might be counterproductive in certain patients with muscle wasting or weakness. In addition to identifying the risks, clinicians also must identify the potential immediate benefits to the patient from any given technique. Some techniques have been shown to be immediately effective in reducing or eliminating certain swallowing deficits (e.g., head turn to compensate for **hemipharyngeal** weakness leading to residue and aspiration). Clinicians should always consider the potential risks of any technique in reference to the potential benefits to the patient.

Functional outcome refers to the long-term benefit of the proposed technique. This is often considered in reference to the goal(s) of therapy. A technique that results in an immediate change in swallowing performance may or may not have a long-term positive impact or it may not be functional for the daily environment. Likewise, some techniques may not have immediate impact, but may produce long-term functional benefit following intensive practice. Therefore choice of technique should be considered in reference to long-term functional outcome, in addition to potential for immediate impact.

Patient empowerment may be interpreted in different ways. One focus of this term is patient involvement in the design of the treatment plan. Involving patients implicates their understanding of the proposed plan of treatment and their willingness to participate in that particular plan. This process makes the patient a partner in treatment rather than only a recipient. Patients who are empowered in this process are known to be more compliant with treatment activities, hence increasing the probabilities for successful outcomes.

OVERVIEW OF TREATMENT OPTIONS FOR DYSPHAGIA

Clinicians should be aware of multiple options for dysphagia intervention, including medical, surgical, and behavioral treatment options. Such knowledge increases pertinent communication with other health care providers and facilitates selection of the best treatment options for individual patients. This section provides a brief overview of some of the more recognized medical, surgical, and behavioral treatment options for dysphagia. Chapter 10 provides a more detailed review of behavioral treatment techniques.

Medical Treatment Options for Dysphagia

Box 9-4 offers an introduction to common medical options for dysphagia intervention. Medical options in this context refer to dietary modifications or pharmacologic management.

Dietary adjustments might seem to be a strange inclusion under medical treatment options; however, clinicians should be aware that diet (oral or non-oral route) may need to be modified to accommodate an underlying disease or condition. Common examples of this are seen in **diabetes** or **hypertension**, both related to stroke. Other examples are found among patients who do not tolerate certain tube feedings well, resulting in diarrhea or constipation. A different example is the patient who requires a minimal (or maximal) amount of caloric intake or hydration for health reasons that may or may not be related to dysphagia. Even if the dietary requirements are tangentially related to the condition contributing to dysphagia, the fact that a specific regimen is required will interact with planning dysphagia intervention.

Pharmacologic management of dysphagia refers to the use of medications to improve some aspect of swallowing function. The most commonly encountered medications are those used to combat reflux, improve gastric motility, and alter secretions. A hierarchy of medications is available to combat reflux symptoms. On the lower end of the hierarchy are approaches such as over-the-counter antacids and certain chewing gum products. The next level of medication is the class of **histamine-receptor antagonists.** These medications are reported to eliminate approximately two thirds of stomach acid. The strongest level of medication is the **proton-pump inhibitor.** These medications are reported to eliminate nearly all stomach acid and represent the strongest pharmacologic approach to acid suppression. Within each class of medications, multiple drugs are available,

Box 9-4	*Common Medical Options for Dysphagia Treatment*

Dietary Modifications	**Pharmacologic Management**
• Special diets	• Antireflux medications
• Regulate nutrition and hydration	• Prokinetic agents
• May interact with feeding route (oral versus nonoral)	• Salivary management

and often choice of medication is based on patient tolerance (fewer side effects) and symptom reduction.

Few medications to improve gastric motility are available. These so-called prokinetic agents are intended to improve esophageal motility, increase lower esophageal sphincter pressure, and promote gastric emptying.

Salivary secretions are important to swallowing functions. They provide important lubrication to the swallowing mechanism and they contain important chemicals that protect the teeth and assist with digestive functions. In general, two components of saliva may be considered. One is the watery saliva that emerges from the sublingual and other salivary glands during chewing or other oral movements. The other is the thicker coating of the internal mucosa. Many medical conditions and medical treatments can alter saliva. Some medical treatments, such as radiotherapy (see Chapter 5), and certain medications reduce the amount of watery saliva, leaving the patient with a dry mouth and complaints of thick, adhering mucus in the mouth and throat. Depending on the cause of the condition, certain medications (**mucolytics**) might be used to thin the thicker secretions, making them easier to swallow (or expectorate if necessary). In addition, certain medications are available that attempt to increase the volume of watery secretions. Alternatively, substances are available (most do not require prescription) that can provide lubrication to the mouth from external application. Medical conditions rarely increase salivary flow. Careful examination of the patient who complains of excessive saliva often reveals a reduction in the frequency of swallowing as the cause for salivary retention in the mouth or pharynx.

Surgical Treatment Options for Dysphagia

Box 9-5 summarizes common surgical interventions for dysphagia. Again, this section is meant to be introductory rather than comprehensive. Three categories of surgical interventions are reviewed: those that improve glottal closure, those that are designed to protect the airway, and those that are designed to improve opening of the pharyngoesophageal segment (PES).

Improving Glottal Closure. Two basic approaches have become popular to improve glottal closure: medialization **thyroplasty** and injection of **biomaterials**. Before these techniques are described, it should be pointed out that it is not always clear which patients will receive swallowing benefit from these procedures.

Box 9-5	*Common Surgical Options for Dysphagia Treatment*

- Improved glottal closure
  —Medialization thyroplasty
  —Injection of biomaterials
- Protection of the airway
  —Stents
  —Laryngotracheal separation
  —Laryngectomy
  —Tracheostomy tubes
  —Feeding tubes

- Improved pharyngoesophageal segment opening
  —Dilatation
  —Myotomy
  —Botulinum toxin injection

Clinical experience has revealed that some patients who aspirate have direct and immediate benefit from improving glottal closure, whereas others receive negligible benefit even in combination with other therapies. In this regard, these techniques should be included within the conceptual background of the dysphagia clinician, but with the caveat that the techniques need to be considered realistically in the context of individual patients.

Medialization thyroplasty is a surgical technique that requires the patient to be sedated but not under general anesthesia. A small incision is made in the lower neck over the thyroid cartilage. A small window is made through the cartilage just behind the vocal fold. The vocal fold is moved toward the midline, and a small piece of medical-grade plastic is placed behind the vocal fold between it and the thyroid cartilage. Because the patient is awake during the procedure, transnasal endoscopy is used to monitor the degree of medialization of the vocal fold, and the patient may be asked to phonate so that the surgeon can assess glottal function for voice production.

Biomaterials may be injected directly into a weakened vocal fold in an attempt to "bulk up" the tissue, thus improving glottal closure. Historically, Teflon was a common material injected into the vocal fold; however, in recent years Teflon has fallen out of favor, being replaced by **autologous fat** (that which is taken from the patient's anterior belly) or **collagen** (commercially available substance). Most commonly (although variations exist), materials are injected into the vocal fold while the patient is under general anesthesia. Typically, injection of biomaterials is used to reduce a smaller glottal gap, whereas medialization thyroplasty is used for larger gaps. However, different surgeons may prefer one technique over the other.

Protecting the Airway. Although glottal closure techniques are intended to enhance airway protection during swallowing, certain medical conditions may require more dramatic airway protection approaches. Some of these surgical approaches are intended for short-term use until a crisis passes, whereas others may be permanent. A laryngeal stent has been described as a "plug" within the larynx to prevent material from entering the airway. Because the glottis is blocked, this procedure requires a tracheostomy. Laryngotracheal separation is a self-describing surgical procedure. The trachea is surgically separated just below the larynx and brought forward to a **tracheostoma**, and the remaining trachea inferior to the larynx is sutured closed. Thus the larynx is in place but is separated from the airway. Both stents and laryngotracheal separation have been described as temporary surgical interventions. A total laryngectomy represents a permanent surgical solution. Although a dramatic (some would say drastic) approach, there are circumstances in which a patient will have better overall function without the larynx. Permanent separation of the air and food tracts may allow the individual to ingest food and liquid safely, and techniques for voice restoration in laryngectomy may facilitate spoken communication.

The use of tracheostomy tubes or feeding tubes in attempts to protect the airway from **prandial aspiration** has been questioned. Available research suggests that this may not be valid reasoning, and that in some patients, tracheostomy tubes can further impair swallowing function and increase the risk of airway compromise. Placement of a feeding tube (nasogastric or gastrostomy) does not necessarily reduce aspiration and may increase the rate and/or severity of aspiration, often from reflux mechanisms. Therefore although both of these surgical options are valid and helpful in individual patients, caution and clear reasoning should be exercised when considering these options.

Improving Pharyngoesophageal Segment Opening. Three general surgical approaches are available to improve opening of the PES: stretching, cutting, or paralyzing. Stretching is accomplished by the process of **dilation.** Dilation may be accomplished by more than one technique, but the process is to stretch the lumen of the PES. If PES opening is restricted by scarring, dilation tears tissue to create a larger opening. However, the risk is twofold: (1) The tear may extend beyond the esophageal tissue, and (2) the effect is often temporary, requiring repeated procedures and, at times, reaching a plateau of benefit. PES limitations resulting from physiologic processes may also respond to dilation. Although dilation is used less often than other techniques, reports have demonstrated benefit from this procedure in cases of physiologic stenosis of the PES.

Surgical myotomy is a technique in which the fibers of the cricopharyngeal muscle within the PES are separated. As with many surgical techniques, variations exist and little evidence suggests that one technique variation is superior to any other. Myotomy may be used in combination with other surgical techniques such as supraglottic laryngectomy or total laryngectomy. Applied judiciously to the appropriate patient, surgical myotomy may provide significant benefit to the dysphagic individual.

Injection of botulinum toxin (Botox) has been described as an effective technique to "relax" the PES. Botulinum toxin works via the process of **chemodenervation,** in which the chemical communication between the motor nerve and the muscle is interrupted. The result is a **paresis** in the muscle. Injection of botulinum toxin has been shown to improve PES opening and hence swallowing function in selected patients. A general rule for selecting patients for this technique (as well as for other techniques focusing on the PES) is that swallowing mechanics above the PES should be optimized. Significant reflux might be considered a contraindication to these techniques.

Behavioral Therapy Options for Dysphagia

More options exist for behavioral interventions for dysphagia than both medical and surgical options combined. Box 9-6 summarizes five general categories of behavioral intervention that may be used in dysphagia intervention. These are meant to be neither exhaustive nor specific (see Chapter 10 for specifics on techniques); rather they are intended to serve as an overview to behavioral therapy approaches.

Box 9-6 *Five General Categories of Behavioral Interventions for Dysphagia*

- Modify the food
- Modify the feeding activity
- Modify the patient
- Modify the swallow
- Modify the mechanism

Modify the Food. Food modifications are among the most widely used behavioral interventions in dysphagia therapy. Food and liquid may be modified in many ways to compensate for a swallowing deficit or in an attempt to alter the swallow pattern toward the goal of improved function. Several aspects of food and liquid modifications may be considered.

Rheology. Modifying the **rheologic** properties of foods and liquids is a common strategy. Thickening liquids with commercial products or purchasing thickened liquids such as nectars is often done in an attempt to slow liquid-bolus transit and form a slightly more cohesive bolus. It is believed that these rheologic changes give patients a better opportunity to swallow without (or with less) airway compromise. This practice has attained a quasi-scientific level at which multiple degrees of thickening have been advocated. Unfortunately, current evidence on the benefits of thickened liquids is limited, and there is some suggestion that patients may not enjoy, and thus may not comply with, a regimen of thickened liquids. Solid foods may also be rheologically modified. A common example of this is pureed food. Experienced clinicians recognize that the concept of puree is highly variable. As one clinician commented, "One man's puree is another man's soup." Nonetheless, clinicians, caregivers, and patients chop, mix, blend, and puree foods to reduce the need for chewing, to reduce the particulate nature of certain foods, and to enhance the ease of swallowing. Another example in this category is the *soft mechanical diet.* This diet level requires mastication, but foods are soft and often form a cohesive bolus when swallowed. A related question is "How soft?" Some patients are able to masticate certain foods with their teeth or tongue without significant reduction in functional eating ability. Little evidence exists that will help formulate guidelines identifying which patients should receive which diet level. Thus clinicians must consider this decision in reference to each individual patient.

Volume. This bolus modification is self-explanatory. Some patients require smaller bolus volumes to be able to control and safely transit the bolus through the swallowing mechanism with minimal postswallow residue. Others may require a larger bolus for various reasons such as increased sensory input. The average bolus size (± 1 standard deviation) of a liquid bolus taken from a cup ranges from 16 to 26 ml and differs between men and women. Bolus volume is one factor that may alter swallow physiology. Thus when small bolus volumes are used, either in assessment or in treatment, swallow physiology may be altered. The important clinical issue is to take all available steps to ascertain that physiology is altered in a positive direction to enhance swallow function.

Temperature. Temperature manipulation is an interesting, multifocal consideration in dysphagia intervention. Cold materials are thought to enhance awareness of a bolus and may have an impact on oropharyngeal swallowing physiology. How cold a bolus should be is an unanswered question. Hot materials (and very cold materials) typically are ingested in smaller amounts and thus may interact with bolus volume. Both hot and cold materials may impact esophageal function. Anyone who has ingested either very hot or very cold materials recognizes the discomfort as that material passes through the esophagus. In **diffuse esophageal spasm**, extreme pain may be triggered by hot or cold materials within the esophagus. The presence of this condition (or other conditions) may be a contraindication for using hot or cold materials in dysphagia intervention.

A different perspective on temperature is that of the patient who does eat by mouth, but inefficiently. These individuals may face the inconvenience and frustration associated with a warm meal getting too cool before the meal is finished. Such patients often report that they use microwaves, ovens, hot plates, or other means to maintain a desired temperature of food over the course of a meal.

Taste and Smell. The senses of taste and smell are not part of the traditional evaluation of swallowing function, and patients are often left to the culinary skills of caregivers or kitchen staff in reference to the palatability of food. However, taste and smell are both essential features of eating. These senses are interrelated, because the four basic tastes are supplemented by flavors (mediated by odor) to provide sensory input during meals. Taste and smell alterations may impact appetite, motivation, and swallowing physiology. Furthermore, taste enhancement (which is typically accomplished by increasing flavor) has been shown to have a positive impact on oral intake in older adults and in certain clinical populations. Hence, taste and smell manipulation may contribute to changes in swallow physiology, appetite, motivation, and enjoyment of meals. The positive aspects of these sensory manipulations may be improved ingestion of food and liquid, contributing to improved health status.

Aesthetics. Figure 9-2 shows photographs of the same pureed meal presented in different aesthetic contexts. In as much as a picture is worth a thousand words, these images should speak loudly.

What a patient sees on a plate might be as important as how it smells or tastes. Certain pureed foods can be visually unappealing and may depress or, at best, not facilitate appetite or motivation to eat. Although aesthetics is still an aspect requiring clinical investigation, available clinical research has focused on enhancing the visual appeal of meals as a factor in improving intake.

Modify the Feeding Activity

Mealtime activity may require modification to accommodate the needs of individual patients. Examples of mealtime modification may include changing the meal schedule, oropharyngeal cleansing or hydration, and/or the use of feeding aids.

For some patients, the meal schedule may be extremely important. For example, the importance of timing meals to the maximal benefit cycle of medications in certain diseases was mentioned in Chapter 4. Other examples include the patient who satiates with small amounts of food and requires multiple meals per day to maintain adequate nutrition. Finally, a common recommendation for timing of oral feedings in patients who are being weaned off feeding tubes is for the patient to ingest the oral meal before tube feeding to take advantage of biologic motivation (hunger) during the oral meals.

Other mealtime adjustments may be warranted in various situations. For example, patients who reside in care facilitates may require special dining

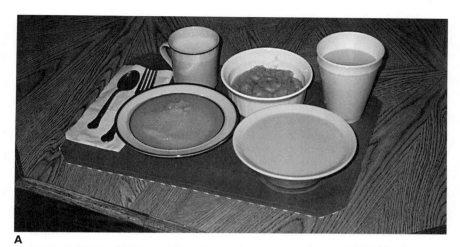

A

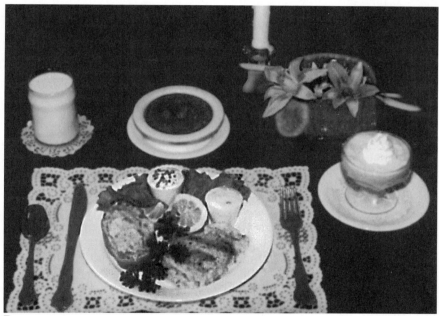

B

FIGURE 9-2 (A) and (B) Photographs of pureed meals with different aesthetic presentation.

arrangements to minimize distractions during meals. These "dysphagia dining rooms" often afford the patient a better caregiver/patient ratio, and thus the potential for increased cueing or other strategies that may facilitate a positive meal experience. This may interact with other mealtime modifications including rate of feeding, specific placement of a bolus, and various clearing strategies to minimize residue and enhance airway protection. During mealtimes, these tactics may be more successful with enhanced clinician or caregiver supervision in an area with reduced distraction.

Patients who experience poor oropharyngeal clearance when swallowing certain foods may benefit from alternating food swallows with liquid swallows. The intent here is to use the subsequent liquid as a "wash" or cleansing mechanism to remove residue from the prior swallow. If a patient has xerostomia (dry mouth), preswallow hydration of the oral cavity may be beneficial. This may be accomplished by swallowing liquid, by sucking on gauze soaked in liquid, by spraying water into the mouth, by using synthetic saliva, or by other methods.

Feeding aids may benefit patients with any number of physiologic or anatomic limitations. Occupational therapists (see Chapter 1) may be invaluable in fashioning devices to accommodate for limitations in hand and limb function. Such devices may be the difference between whether the patient is an independent self-feeder or a dependent feeder. Other modifications may be required in cases of trauma or surgical restructuring of the oral mechanism. Possible alternatives may include the use of nipples, flow-controlled feeders, straws, specialized utensils (e.g., glossectomy spoons), or catheters.

Modify the Patient

The most common strategies used in this category are positioning strategies. These might involve head-position strategies such as head-turn or chin-tuck maneuvers or whole body–positioning strategies. Chapter 10 addresses head-position strategies in more detail. This section addresses whole body positioning.

An initial caveat is the reminder that for certain patients, changing body position may require the consultation of other dysphagia team members, specifically the physical therapist (see Chapter 1). In general, the patient should be positioned such that physical capabilities are maximized and accommodations to improve swallowing can be incorporated. With that in mind, common position adjustments might include the patient tilting to the side or back, side-lying, or maintaining an upright posture.

Patients with hemipharyngeal weakness may benefit from tilting the upper body such that the stronger side is lower and able to benefit from gravity to assist bolus transit. This positioning technique may be combined with a head turn toward the weaker side of the pharynx. An exaggerated example of this approach is the side-lying position. This technique may be used in circumstances in which patients want to maximize residual pharyngeal muscle function, while at the same time reducing bolus speed by removing the influence of gravity. If pharyngeal asymmetry exists, the stronger side is typically lower.

Tilting the patient backward may be beneficial in cases in which oral movements reduce transit of the bolus through the mouth or in which significant residue remains in the piriform sinuses following a swallow. One consideration for this technique should be airway protection ability.

Upright posture may be an important consideration in patients with oropharyngeal or esophageal deficits. Residue in the proximal esophagus may reflux into the hypopharynx during or after meals. Keeping the patient upright adds the potential protective mechanism of gravity in an attempt to minimize the upward movement of esophageal residue. In cases of severe reflux, upright posture during and after meals may be important even if the patient receives nutrition from a gastrostomy tube. Finally, it is well known that elevating the head of the bed is beneficial in combating nocturnal reflux.

Modify the Mechanism

Attempts to modify the swallowing mechanism might include motor exercises, sensory stimulation, and prosthetic adjustments to compensate for physiologic or anatomic deficits. Motor exercises typically address one of five features of motor function: strength, range, tone, steadiness, or accuracy. Depending on the underlying disease and the overt movement dysfunction, various techniques may be applied. Common approaches to improve strength may include resistance activities, in which the patient attempts to move against resistance. Range of movement may be increased by stretching activities. An example of this is the stretching activities used by patients with **trismus** in an attempt to increase mouth opening. Accuracy and steadiness impact coordination. Again depending on the specific attributes of the movement dysfunction, various techniques may be used, ranging from altering the rheologic properties of swallowed materials to using a contained bolus that is manipulated around the mouth but not swallowed (this occasionally is referred to with the charming name *chew bag*).

Sensory stimulation activities may involve changes in taste, temperature, or the application of pressure. Limited experimentation has occurred with the use of electrical stimulation as a sensory approach to improving movement associated with swallowing. Finally, improved oral hygiene, when indicated, may facilitate improved sensory functions and reduce disease risks.

Prosthetic management may be accomplished in conjunction with a maxillofacial prosthodontist as a member of the dysphagia team. Prosthodontists can fabricate palatal lifts, obturators, and other devices to fill anatomic deviations that might exist in certain patients with dysphagia.

Modify the Swallow

Swallow modifications focus primarily on altering the physiology of the attempted swallow. These activities often require active participation from the patient and intensive practice to induce movement change. Chapter 10 provides a detailed review of the more common behavioral techniques to modify swallow physiology.

FRAMEWORK FOR MAKING TREATMENT DECISIONS

Many approaches may be followed in developing intervention plans. The following section offers a framework detailing steps in clinical decision making that may be helpful to dysphagia clinicians. Three aspects are considered: (1) sources of information used in treatment planning, (2) forming meaningful clinical questions, and (3) developing individual treatment plans.

Sources of Information Used in Treatment Planning

Figure 9-3 presents a flowchart detailing potential sources of clinical information that may address treatment issues. In this depiction, treatment issues are divided into "independence issues" and "safety issues." Independence issues include supervision, assistance, and compliance. *Supervision* refers to the patient's need for direct supervision during mealtime, perhaps to monitor food intake and use of compensations or for other reasons. *Assistance* refers to the use of direct physical assistance during mealtime. *Compliance* refers to the patient's adherence to an intervention plan. Safety issues include airway protection and nutrition and hydration. *Airway protection* refers to the overt presence of aspiration or the risk of aspiration from excessive residue or other factors. This term should also consider airway obstruction from solid foods. *Nutrition and hydration* refer to the patient's ability to ingest sufficient calories and fluids. Independence and safety issues often interact. For example, the patient who requires but does not receive adequate assistance may have reduced airway protection or may ingest insufficient amounts of food or liquid.

The diagram depicted in Figure 9-3 attempts to estimate from where assessment information relative to independence and safety issues is derived. Independence issues may be addressed more from the physical examination and the feeding examination. Instrumental examinations may not be needed to address independence issues. Conversely, instrumental examinations seem essential in making safety determinations, especially airway protection issues. Nutrition and hydration issues are better addressed through a combination of the instrumental examination and the feeding examination.

Forming Meaningful Clinical Questions

Once relevant clinical information has been gathered and organized into some conceptual framework (such as that depicted in Figure 9-3), a next logical step is to pose the question, "Which treatment technique(s) are best suited to this individual patient or problem?" This becomes part of an **evidence-based**

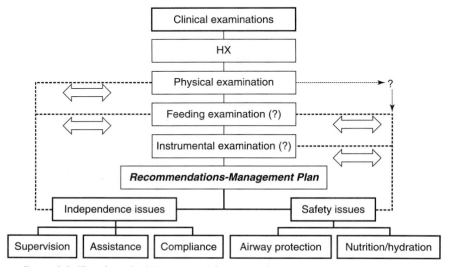

Figure 9-3 Flowchart depicting potential sources of treatment planning information based on various components of the dysphagia evaluation.

approach to treatment of dysphagia. The schematic depicted in Figure 9-4 offers one potential framework from which to formulate meaningful clinical questions pertaining to treatment options.

Starting with the focus on the patient or problem, clinicians should first frame the question. In the example in Figure 9-4, a patient with neurogenic pharyngeal dysphagia resulting from nonprogressive disease is presented. This patient demonstrates residue and aspiration on examination. Based on the examination, a treatment option is considered—in this case, the use of sEMG biofeedback. Next, treatment alternatives are considered—in this case, teaching the Mendelsohn maneuver in isolation. Finally, expected outcomes are framed as a question. Can the use of biofeedback in addition to the clinical maneuver improve functional outcome (e.g., better swallow) while reducing the number of treatment sessions (i.e., increasing efficiency of therapy)? After forming this question, clinicians need to survey the evidence on these techniques to find the answer. For this specific example, evidence supporting the use of biofeedback would be research indicating that use of this technique enhanced functional outcomes of therapy with less time investment than therapy without this technique. If such evidence was identified, the clinician should consider using this technique.

Planning Individual Therapy Strategies

Once the treatment question is formulated and treatment options have been systematically considered (based on available evidence), the individual treatment plan may be developed. One format for the treatment plan is depicted in Box 9-7. *Goals* are statements of anticipated outcome based on the patient's pretreatment functional level with consideration of the clinical examination results (presumably identifying some or all of the reasons for the pretreatment functional level). Beginning clinicians are encouraged to keep in mind that goals can change as the patient's status changes. In addition, it may be beneficial clinical practice to focus on a single functional goal, especially in the

Focus Your Question	Starting with your patient, ask: "How would I describe a group of similar patients?"	Ask: "Which technique am I considering?"	Ask: "What is the main alternative or option?"	Ask: "What can I hope to gain?"
		Be specific	Be specific	Be specific
Example	In patients with neurogenic pharyngeal dysphagia in nonprogressive disease with residue and aspiration....	"Would use sEMG biofeedback"	"Compared with only a Mendelsohn maneuver"	"Improve the functional outcome of therapy and decrease the number of therapy sessions"

FIGURE 9-4 One framework from which to pose meaningful clinical questions regarding best treatment options.

Box 9-7   *One Format for Developing Individual Treatment Plans for Dysphagia*

Goals
- Statement(s) of anticipated functional outcome

Objectives
- Target aspects of the swallow and/or patient that require change to reach the functional goal

Action Plans
- Activities in which the patient and clinician engage; procedures and progress monitors to be used in therapy are specified

---

initial aspects of therapy. Goals should be simple statements that are understood by the patient and caregivers. For example, a goal statement for a patient who is taking no food or liquid by mouth may be "to establish the safe and consistent oral intake of any substance in any amount." Conceptually, if the patient cannot reach this functional level, further advances in oral intake are unlikely. Setting goals that are too ambitious may reduce patient (and clinician) motivation and compliance with a treatment program. Surpassing goals most likely will not contribute to that scenario.

Objectives target those items regarding the swallow and/or the patient that require change for the functional goal to be reached. These may be specific aspects of swallow physiology such as increased hyolaryngeal elevation or patient-related aspects such as rate of eating. If objectives are met, goals will be reached.

Action plans reflect those activities in which the patient and/or clinician will engage. These are direct statements of procedures. They should include instructions to the patient reflecting technique, frequency of practice, amount to be swallowed, or other directly overt aspects of the therapy program. In addition, action plans should include techniques to monitor the immediate impact of the treatment technique(s). These monitors do not need to be elaborate, nor do they require repeated instrumental examinations to evaluate progress. However, often based on instrumental examinations, monitors may be behaviors that indicate change in the swallow performance. For example, consider the patient who expectorates following each swallowing attempt. One potential monitor of performance change in swallowing might be a reduction in the frequency of postswallow expectoration. Actions plans impact objectives that in turn impact functional goals and hence overt swallowing performance.

Framework for Planning Treatment

Figures 9-5 and 9-6 depict one organizational framework for planning dysphagia treatment. Using pharyngeal dysphagia as an example, these flowcharts present the general organization of the treatment planning concepts depicted in this chapter, followed by a specific clinical example.

At the top of the hierarchy (see Figure 9-5), pretreatment functional level is determined. As indicated previously in this chapter, severity of dysphagia

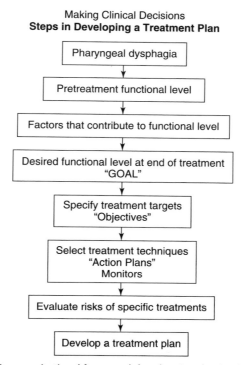

Making Clinical Decisions
Steps in Developing a Treatment Plan

Pharyngeal dysphagia

↓

Pretreatment functional level

↓

Factors that contribute to functional level

↓

Desired functional level at end of treatment
"GOAL"

↓

Specify treatment targets
"Objectives"

↓

Select treatment techniques
"Action Plans"
Monitors

↓

Evaluate risks of specific treatments

↓

Develop a treatment plan

FIGURE 9-5 An organizational framework for planning dysphagia treatment.

or functional level is a complex issue. One perspective might be to consider the amount and type of food and liquid a patient is safely ingesting by mouth at the time of evaluation. Although simplistic, this approach may be the most meaningful to the patient. Extending from this functional level are those swallowing factors believed to be contributing to the reduced function. Next, a goal for therapy is established. This is an outcome statement and, whenever possible, it should be developed in conjunction with the patient and/or caregivers. Objectives and specific actions are selected as stepping stones by which the patient may reach the functional goal. Finally, risks of the respective treatment techniques are considered in reference to the anticipated benefit(s).

In Figure 9-6A the example of pharyngeal dysphagia is used, and specific decisions that might be made during the planning process are detailed. Early in the planning process, the clinician must decide if the patient is a good candidate for therapy. This involves a prognosis. Several considerations for treatment candidacy were discussed earlier in this chapter; however, prognosis for therapy response is not an exact science for dysphagia. The best course of action may be to overtly recognize the basis for any prognostic decision based on available evidence.

If the patient is thought to be a good therapy candidate, goals and objectives are developed. Figure 9-6A presents four objectives that may be considered in

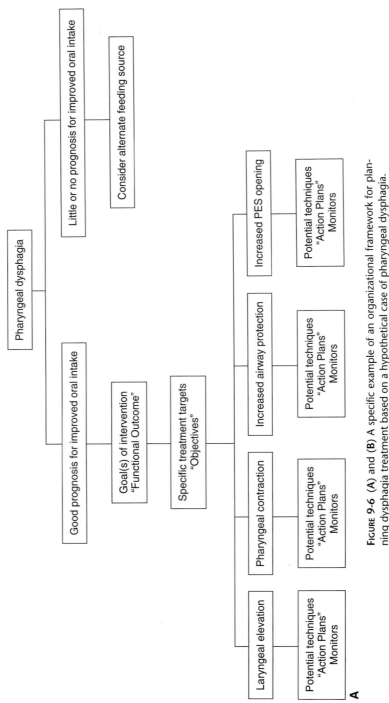

Figure 9-6 **(A)** and **(B)** A specific example of an organizational framework for planning dysphagia treatment based on a hypothetical case of pharyngeal dysphagia.

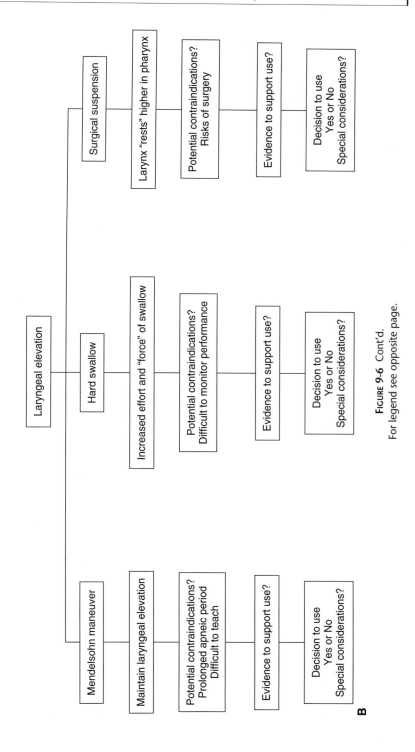

FIGURE 9-6 Cont'd.
For legend see opposite page.

pharyngeal dysphagia: laryngeal elevation, pharyngeal contraction, airway protection, and PES opening. The next step is to select action plans for each of these objectives. Figure 9-6B takes one of the objectives, laryngeal elevation, and considers three potential action plans. The Mendelsohn maneuver facilitates sustained laryngeal elevation and thus is an appropriate action plan. On the negative side, this maneuver may prolong the apneic pause during swallowing and thus may be contraindicated for some patients with compromised respiratory function. In addition, it is difficult to teach this maneuver to certain patients. Clinicians should consider the available evidence supporting use of this maneuver for the specific problem and patient under consideration (see Chapter 10). Finally, the decision to use or not to use a technique is made along with any special considerations. An example of a special consideration for this maneuver is using biofeedback to assist in teaching what may be a difficult maneuver to teach. Similar considerations apply to the "hard swallow" technique and to the surgical technique laryngeal suspension. The clinician must consider the following questions: What is the intended impact of the technique? Are there any potential contraindications or risks? Is there any available evidence to support use of the technique?

TAKE HOME NOTES

- Primary considerations for dysphagia treatment include airway protection and nutrition and hydration. These may be influenced by multiple factors related to the patient, the underlying disease or disorder, the clinician, and/or the health care environment.
- Dysphagia treatment is often multifocal and multidisciplinary. Clinicians should be familiar with multiple treatment options across medical, surgical, and behavioral domains.
- Choice of a specific therapy technique may depend on the specifics of the patient's health care status, the skills of the treating clinician, the health care environment, or other factors.
- Clinicians must make sure to evaluate health care risks and potential obstacles when considering treatment options.
- A comprehensive therapy plan should include a statement of functional goals, objectives to meet those goals, and specific actions to initiate for each objective.

CASE EXAMPLE

A 78-year-old woman who is 6 months post–left cerebrovascular accident and who has no known family is now residing in a long-term care facility. She has a possible history of a prior stroke, but no details are available. She is ambulatory with a walker and physical assistance; however, she spends most waking hours in a wheelchair or in bed. She is currently on a total oral diet, which is modified to puree and thickened liquids. She is a self-feeder. She was referred for dysphagia evaluation and treatment secondary to continuing weight loss and reports of coughing during meals. A review of her chart indicates recent history of repeated urinary tract infections.

Clinical examination reveals a small woman who is interactive but with subtle signs of impaired mental status and a possible mild aphasia. She demonstrated no overt corticobulbar deficits. The right arm and leg are paretic, with the leg being more involved than the arm. When asked about swallowing, she replied that she swallows "just fine." When asked about the food at the facility, she indicated that it is "okay."

Fluoroscopic swallowing evaluation indicated mild physiologic deviations including slow oral transit, reduced hyolaryngeal elevation, reduced pharyngeal contraction, and reduced PES opening. Postswallow residue was noted in the valleculae and the piriform recesses, primarily on thicker materials. When liquid was used to remove residue, a minute amount of aspiration was noted postswallow. The patient demonstrated a consistent reactive cough with aspiration. Maneuvers such as the chin tuck or head turn had no impact on this pattern of swallowing. The patient was able to chew a cracker, but had difficulty forming a cohesive oral bolus and removing the material from her mouth.

Considerations for Treatment Planning The first consideration for treatment planning is the current functional eating level of the patient. In this particular case, the patient is taking all food and liquid by mouth but with a restricted diet of puree and thickened liquids. She is a self-feeder. A primary concern is continuing weight loss. A related concern might be the recurring urinary tract infections.

The next consideration is that of factors that may contribute to the existing functional level. Both the weight loss and the recurring infections may relate to an insufficient intake of nutrition and hydration. This is a point to address through communication with the long-term care facility. Predisposing factors may not always be overt and clear, so many issues should be considered. A few factors to consider in this case include swallow physiology, physical status, appetite, and the patient's environment. The clinician must consider the functional eating level in reference to the observed swallow physiology as seen fluoroscopically. This patient demonstrated slow transit and mild reduction in pharyngeal components of the swallow. She had more difficulty with dry, particulate materials (cracker). She did aspirate mildly in certain circumstances and had a strong reactive cough. This last observation may relate to the observed coughing during meals. The relationship of the physiologic deviations to the functional eating pattern is more difficult to understand. Overall slowness may be related to prolonged mealtimes and thus to reduced food intake. Is it possible that this patient is demonstrating mild cognitive changes that may reflect early-stage dementia and the swallowing changes that may accompany the cognitive change (see Chapter 4)? This might be one area for further clinical examination. Are there other possibilities that may help support or refute a possible relationship between the observed swallow physiology and the functional eating pattern? Physical status may help explain some of the reduced intake of food and liquid. Recall that this patient is a self-feeder. In addition, recall that she has some weakness in the right upper limb and may have had a previous stroke. It would be beneficial to observe her eating a meal to help determine the extent to which physical limitation may restrict intake of food and liquid. Appetite loss may be another factor in reduced intake. Although the patient described the food as "okay," she did not indicate high motivation for eating. This may be related to cognitive or environmental (social) issues. Depression should also be considered. The current dining situation may be distracting, noisy, or unpleasant to the patient. She may require cues to continue eating or other adjustments that are not provided in her current situation. Under these circumstances, she may have reduced intake. All of these factors must be considered to derive the best possible intervention for this patient.

The primary goal for this patient might be to stop weight loss and subsequently to increase weight to appropriate levels. A related goal may be to reduce urinary tract infections (if these result from reduced hydration). To address these goals, the factors contributing to the current functional level must be addressed, and treatment objectives must be selected for those factors that may be altered to improve functional status. One obvious objective is to increase the amount of nutrition and hydration taken by mouth. The methods by which this is accomplished should relate directly to those factors perceived to contribute to reduced oral intake.

Selecting specific action plans in this particular case may require a period of further observation under differing conditions. For example, it might be prudent to observe this patient eating a more rheologically complex meal, to observe her eating meals of varying amounts, to enhance taste properties, to increase mealtime cues, and/or to change the dining environment. The best intervention approach may be a combination of these strategies. One monitor for improvement might be the amount of calories and hydration consumed daily. The functional outcome would be weight gain to appropriate levels and reduced urinary tract infections.

CHAPTER TERMS

apneic pause a temporary stoppage of respiration during swallowing

autologous fat fat taken from the patient (typically from the anterior belly) and injected into the patient's vocal fold

biomaterials a general term referring to materials that may be placed within the body

chemodenervation interruption of nerve function by a chemical agent

collagen a fibrous protein material found in connective tissue including skin, tendons, and ligaments

diabetes a general term referring to diseases marked by excessive urination; commonly referring to diabetes mellitus, which results from inadequate production or use of insulin

diffuse esophageal spasm a condition marked by generalized spasm in the esophagus, usually resulting in significant retrosternal pain

dilation expanding an opening with a dilator (the term dilatation is also used to describe the same procedure)

evidence-based approach the conscientious use of current best evidence in making decisions about the care of individual patients

hemipharyngeal pertaining to half of the pharynx, usually referring to a deficit in the right or left aspect of the pharynx

histamine-receptor antagonists medications that block the stimulation of cells by histamine (used to reduce gastric acid secretion); also known as *histamine-blocking agents*

hypertension higher than normal blood pressure

mucolytics medications that reduce the viscosity of saliva

paresis weakness; partial or incomplete paralysis

prandial aspiration passage of food or liquid material into the upper airway during meals *proton-pump inhibitors* medications that reduce gastric acid secretion to a greater degree than do histamine-blocking agents

rheologic pertaining to the study of the deformation and flow of materials

thyroplasty a surgical procedure in which a window is cut in the thyroid cartilage for medialization of the vocal fold underlying the cartilage

tracheostoma an opening into the trachea through the neck

trismus tonic contraction of the muscles of mastication contributing to reduced mouth opening

SUGGESTED READINGS

Adnerhill I, Eckberg O, Groher ME: Determining normal bolus size for thin liquids, *Dysphagia* 4:1, 1989.

Ali GN et al: Predictors of outcome following cricopharyngeal disruption for pharyngeal dysphagia, *Dysphagia* 12:133, 1997.

Cichero J et al: How thick is thick? Multicenter study of the rheological and material property characteristics of mealtime fluids and videofluoroscopy fluids, *Dysphagia* 15:188, 2000.

de Carle DJ: Gastro-oesophageal reflux disease, *Med J Aust* 169:549, 1998.

Hillel AD et al: Amyotrophic lateral sclerosis severity scale, *Neuroepidemiology* 8: 142, 1989.

Hoebler C et al: Particle size of solid food after human mastication and in vitro simulation of oral breakdown, *Int J Food Sci Nutr* 51:353, 2000.

Isshiki N: Progress in laryngeal framework surgery, *Acta Otolaryngol* 120:120, 2000.

Kelly JH: Management of upper esophageal sphincter disorders: indications and complications of myotomy, *Am J Med* 108(Suppl):43S, 2000.

Leonard RJ et al: Structural displacements in normal swallowing: a videofluoroscopic study, *Dysphagia* 15:146, 2000.

List MA, Ritter-Sterr C, Lansky SB: A performance status scale for head and neck cancer patients, *Cancer* 66:564, 1990.

Musson ND et al: Nature, nurture, nutrition: interdisciplinary programs to address the prevention of malnutrition and dehydration, *Dysphagia* 5:96, 1990.

O'Neil KH et al: The dysphagia outcome and severity scale, *Dysphagia* 14:139, 1999.

Pardoe EM: Development of a multistage diet for dysphagia, *J Am Diet Assoc* 93: 568, 1993.

Robinson M: Medical management of gastroesophageal reflux disease. In Castell D, Richter J, editors: *The esophagus*, ed 3, New York, 1999, Lippincott-Raven.

Rosen CA: Phonosurgical vocal fold injection: procedures and materials, *Otolaryngol Clin North Am* 33:1087, 2000.

Schiffman SS: Intensification of sensory properties of foods for the elderly, *J Nutr* 130(Suppl):927S, 2000.

Scolapio JS et al: Dysphagia without endoscopically evident disease: to dilate or not? *Am J Gastroenterol* 96:327, 2001.

Shanley C, O'Loughlin G: Dysphagia among nursing home residents: an assessment and management protocol, *J Gerontol Nurs* 26:35, 2000.

Storr M, Allescher HD: Esophageal pharmacology and treatment of primary motility disorders, *Dis Esophagus* 12:241, 1999.

Westergren A et al: Eating difficulties, complications and nursing interventions during a period of three months after a stroke, *J Adv Nurs* 35:416, 2001.

CHAPTER 10

Overview of Behavioral Treatment Strategies

FOCUS QUESTIONS

1   What is evidence-based practice? Discuss how it might be used to make treatment decisions for dysphagia.
2   What are some of the basic differences between compensatory techniques and rehabilitative techniques? How does this distinction apply to specific therapy techniques?
3   What impact do various therapy techniques have on the swallowing mechanism?
4   What are the expected functional benefits associated with various behavioral treatment strategies?

EVIDENCE-BASED PRACTICE

In the late 1990s, the Dutch Neurological Society presented guidelines for treatment of dysphagia in acute stroke. These guidelines were critical of existing practices, claiming that no scientific evidence existed to justify the use of video-fluoroscopy in the evaluation of dysphagia nor to justify swallowing therapy or diet modification in the treatment of dysphagia. This scenario raised critical questions concerning dysphagia management, both in acute stroke and in general. What is the evidence that supports the use of swallowing therapy for dysphagia? To address this question, a basic understanding of evidence-based practice is required.

Definitions of Evidence-Based Practice

Many overlapping definitions of evidence-based practice exist. Most share similar concepts and vary primarily in the presentation of those concepts. Evidence-based practice is the conscientious, explicit, and judicious use of current best evidence in making decisions about the care of individual patients. Note the focus on *individual patients* in this definition. This focus is an important concept in evidence-based practice. Other definitions refer to the fact that evidence-based practice is based on best current evidence that begins and ends with caring for patients. Another variation refers to the use of simple rules of logic and science to appraise and apply evidence from research to the care of individual patients. Finally, evidence-based practice has been described as the process of finding, evaluating, and using the best available evidence to inform and improve clinical practice.

Common concepts in these definitions are the focus on the individual patient and the acquisition, evaluation, and use of scientific information to improve the level of care provided to individual patients. Principles of evidence-based practice may apply to the entire spectrum of clinical practice, from the accuracy of diagnostic tests, to prognosis, to the **efficacy** and safety of rehabilitation and prevention efforts.

Levels of Evidence

Clinical practitioners may obtain information relative to patient care from various sources. Some information sources include the following: prior personal experience (it worked before so I will try it again), textbooks (although these are rarely opened once the course is completed), expert advice either directly or through continuing education courses (eminence value—if the experts say it, it must be true), professional practice guidelines (hopefully based on best evidence, but not always), commercial sales people ("This product is just what you need"), and journal articles (although research has shown that the frequency of professional reading declines proportionately with years away from university). An important distinction is the difference between information and evidence. Evidence results from a controlled approach to the study of clinical questions. The strength of the evidence directly relates to the strength or degree of control in the studies used to address clinical questions. Box 10-1 presents one system for evaluating the strength of evidence based on the design of research studies producing that evidence. Box 10-2 includes definitions of the various types of research studies that compose the respective levels of evidence. Most current evidence in support of behavioral treatment in dysphagia is based

---

Box 10-1   *One Classification of Strength of Evidence in Clinical Research*

Stronger Evidence

Level I
A. Systematic review of multiple randomized, controlled trials (RCTs)
B. Large RCT with clear-cut results

Level II
A. Small RCT with uncertain results
B. Systematic review of cohort studies
C. Individual cohort study

Level III
A. Systematic review of case-control studies
B. Individual case-control study

Level IV
A. Case series with historical controls
B. Case series without historical controls
C. Poor case-control and cohort studies

Level V
A. Expert opinion (eminence value)
B. Critical review based on physiology (biologic plausibility)

Weaker Evidence

on small cohort studies, case-controlled studies, historical-controlled studies, or outcomes research. Stronger evidence in the form of randomized, controlled trials is emerging in certain patient subgroups.

Questions Related to Applying Evidence

Once the type of study and hence level of evidence has been identified, a series of pragmatic questions might be addressed to determine whether a given technique is applicable in a given clinical practice setting. Such questions might address the technique, patient issues, outcome issues, and clinician readiness.

It is imperative to understand the technique to consider its application in clinical practice. A basic question is whether published articles, presentations, or other sources of information provide clear descriptions or instructions on how to perform the technique under consideration. This information might incorporate a clear description of the technique and specific instructions for how to apply the technique clinically, including how often and under what conditions the technique should be used. It is important to identify whether the published evidence was gathered from a group of patients similar to the patient being considered for a given technique. For example, evidence supporting the use of a given technique

---

| **Box 10-2** | *Definitions of Study Designs Used to Evaluate Strength of Evidence in Clinical Research* |

Case Series

Reports on a number of patients receiving the same treatment. May involve historical comparisons, which could be a group of patients treated before the treatment of interest was available or the historical performance of the patients in the series before receiving the treatment of interest.

Case-Control Study

Often a retrospective study of patients with a specific disease or outcome of interest compared with a group of similar patients without the disease or outcome of interest. This might involve looking at specific outcomes in a group of patients who received a treatment compared with a similar (individually matched) group of patients who did not receive that treatment.

Cohort Study

An observational study in which a group of similar patients may or may not receive a treatment based on their individual circumstances (natural selection). Outcomes are observed following treatment, typically over an extended period.

Randomized, Controlled Trial

Also called a *randomized clinical trial,* this design requires random assignment of patients into a treatment group and a control group. Both groups are treated exactly the same way with the exception of the treatment of interest.

Systematic Review

The systematic evaluation of evidence across multiple clinical trials. When the review uses special statistical methods to combine the results of several studies, it is called a *metaanalysis.*

Box 10-3	*Questions That May Apply to the Selection of Therapy Techniques for Dysphagia*

Are the patients in the study similar to my patient?
- Clinical profile
- Imaging studies (endoscopy/fluoroscopy)
- Acute or chronic and clinical environment

Was the therapy technique adequately described?
- Stated purpose
- Clear instructions
- How and when to apply and when to stop
- Patient role versus clinician role

Do I have the clinical skills and technology to use this technique?
- Feasibility in my practice
- Specific knowledge or technology
- Specific training available

Were the outcomes similar to those that I want to achieve for my patient?
- Amount of oral intake
- Type of food
- Physiologic changes

Were failures reported?
- Why did some patients fail with this technique?

---

for stroke patients may not be applicable to patients with head/neck cancer. Another consideration might be what the technique is intended to accomplish. Compensations are considered short-term adjustments that facilitate improved swallowing but do not have a lasting impact on swallow physiology. If a compensatory technique is not used, the patient is not expected to swallow successfully. Rehabilitation techniques are anticipated to enact lasting changes in swallowing performance that will remain even after use of the technique is discontinued. Given this distinction, clinicians may ask whether a technique is intended to change the swallow physiology, to accommodate various bolus characteristics, to have short- or long-term impact, or to have other influences on the patient or the swallow mechanism. Several treatment technique considerations were addressed in Chapter 9. These considerations relate to how a given technique fits into a plan of care, whether a technique should be applied in isolation or in combination, and how the technique relates to the anticipated outcome of treatment. Clinicians should also ask whether they have received the appropriate training and whether they hold the appropriate skills to apply a given technique. Box 10-3 summarizes some of the more salient questions that might be appropriate in evaluating techniques for use in dysphagia treatment.

WHICH TECHNIQUES AND WHAT TO CONSIDER

Box 10-4 lists therapy techniques that have been described in dysphagia treatment literature. Each of these techniques has some degree of supporting evidence

Box 10-4	*List of Therapy Techniques Discussed in This Chapter*

- Postural adjustments
  — Body posture
  — Head posture
- Supraglottic swallow
- Super supraglottic swallow
- Mendelsohn maneuver

- Effortful swallow
- Tongue hold or Masako maneuver
- Isotonic/isometric exercise:
  Shaker exercise
- Thermal-tactile application
- Adjunctive biofeedback

in subgroups of patients with dysphagia. The following information is presented (if available) for each technique: (1) description of the technique including intended or anticipated impact on swallowing mechanism and function, (2) impact on swallow physiology in normal and abnormal swallowing, and (3) outcomes in clinical application.

General Postural Adjustments

Postural adjustments may involve the entire body or only the head. In general, changes in head and/or body posture have been shown to be effective in reducing aspiration in various patient groups. The reasoning for this may be that changes in posture redirect the bolus and may change the speed of bolus flow, giving the patient more time to adjust the swallow. Typically, body posture changes involve lying down and/or side-lying. Both of these positions are expected to reduce the impact of gravity either during the swallow or on postswallow residue. The side-lying technique may be applied when a difference in pharyngeal function is noted between the right and left sides. In this situation, conventional wisdom suggests that the stronger side be the down side. This makes use of gravity to direct the bolus (or residue) toward the stronger hemipharynx.

Body postural adjustments are considered compensatory, in that they (hopefully) are used for a specified period until swallowing functions can improve. The immediate impact of postural adjustments may be examined during instrumental imaging studies such as fluoroscopy or endoscopy. However, in some situations, these techniques may be needed long term. For example, in patients with severe physical impairment, body posture adjustments may be required for an extended period to maintain safety during swallowing.

Postural adjustments may not be the ideal intervention for patients who are at risk for **noncompliance** because of physical or cognitive limitations. In addition, change in body posture may impact esophageal motor functions. The impact of body posture changes on esophageal function should be examined in patients with signs of esophageal deficit.

A different application for body posture changes is seen in the patient with reflux disease or with poor esophageal motility. Patients with severe reflux (even those being fed through a tube) may benefit from maintaining an upright posture during and after feeding. This may help reduce or prevent reflux that may contribute to aspiration. In addition, nocturnal head-of-bed elevation has long been advocated for patients with nocturnal reflux. This simple postural adjustment has been shown to be highly effective in promoting acid clearance from the esophagus.

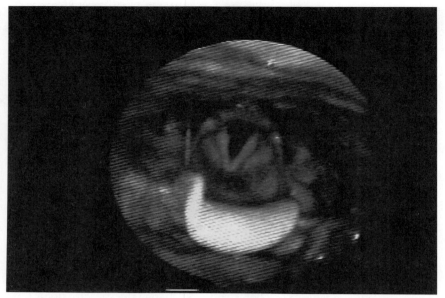

FIGURE 10-1 Oropharyngeal widening resulting from head extension (chin raise). This photo was taken from a video.

Head Postural Adjustments

Changes in head posture may include extension, flexion, or rotation. Head extension may be accomplished by raising the chin. This has the anatomic effect of widening the oropharynx (Figure 10-1) and may be helpful in moving a bolus from the mouth into the pharynx when oral or lingual deficits are present. Head extension may also impact the pharyngoesophageal segment (PES), specifically creating increased **intraluminal** pressure and decreased duration of relaxation in the PES. These changes may complicate an existing swallowing problem. Furthermore, head extension has been shown to reduce laryngeal closure in both healthy adults and those with dysphagia. Thus although head extension may be a useful clinical technique in patients with difficulty transporting a bolus from the mouth to the pharynx, it may contribute to swallowing difficulties in patients who have airway protection or PES deficits.

Head flexion has been shown to facilitate improved airway protection in patients who demonstrate deficits in airway protection during swallowing. Flexing the head (chin tuck) has the anatomic effect of narrowing the oropharynx, as shown in Figure 10-2, and reducing the distance between the hyoid bone and the larynx. The physiologic effects of head flexion have been reported to include weaker pharyngeal contraction during swallowing. Thus this technique may not be well used in patients with pharyngeal weakness. At least one study concluded that this postural maneuver was not useful for patients who demonstrated delay in swallow initiation and postswallow residual in the piriform recesses. Another report suggested that this technique might not be maximally effective for patients with PES dysfunction or with

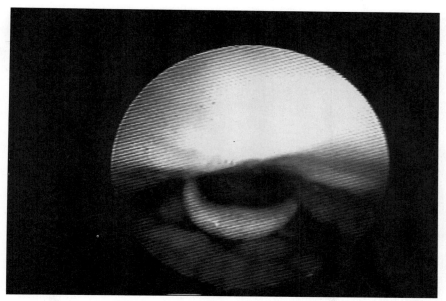

FIGURE 10-2 Oropharyngeal narrowing resulting from head flexion (chin tuck). This photo was taken from a video.

multiple swallow deficits. Finally, this technique may need to be combined with other strategies, including other postures or bolus changes, to produce maximal benefit. Because this is such a simple task to perform, it may be evaluated quickly during instrumental studies.

The chin-tuck maneuver is considered compensatory. It is typically introduced as a temporary adjustment to increase airway protection during swallowing. Before using this technique as a therapy strategy, its functional benefit should be verified during an imaging study. Long-term rehabilitative effects have not yet been reported for this technique.

Head rotation, or the head-turn maneuver, also has been used as a treatment technique. This technique has been advocated primarily in cases of unilateral pharyngeal deficit. Conventional wisdom suggests that patients turn the head toward the weaker side in cases of hemilateral impairment. The anatomic result of this postural maneuver is a narrowing or closing off of the swallowing tract on the side toward which the head is turned. This effect is demonstrated in Figure 10-3, in which the head is turned to each side with the corresponding change in oropharyngeal configuration. This closure effect may not extend throughout the hypopharynx, but may be restricted to the level of the hyoid bone at the superior hypopharynx, leaving the inferior aspects of this area open in some patients. Physiologic effects of head rotation include a drop in PES pressure and a corresponding increase in PES opening. This is anticipated to facilitate an increase in the amount swallowed, with less residue and reduced risk of airway compromise.

Like many postural maneuvers, head rotation may be considered a compensatory technique, not a life-long adjustment in swallowing. In addition, like

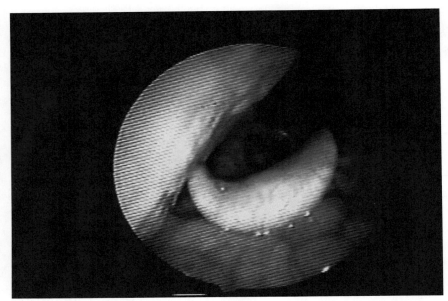

A

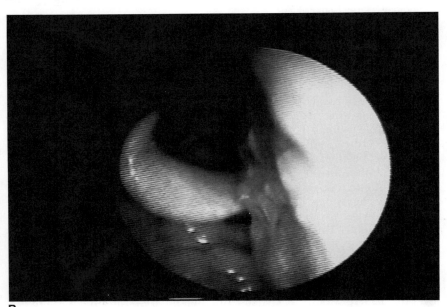

B

FIGURE 10-3 Changes in oropharyngeal configuration resulting from head rotation. **(A)** Right. **(B)** Left. These photos were taken from video.

other techniques in this category, effectiveness may be reduced by cognitive **(compliance)** factors, by physical factors, or by the presence of multiple swallowing deficits. Finally, the functional effects of a head-turn maneuver may be checked easily during imaging studies.

Protecting the Airway: Supraglottic and Super Supraglottic Swallows

The supraglottic swallow and super supraglottic swallow maneuvers are techniques designed to protect the airway from aspiration of food and liquid by closing the airway before swallowing and then coughing immediately after the swallow to clear any residue that may be on the vocal folds. The difference between these related maneuvers is the degree of effort in the preswallow breath-hold. As implied by the name, the super supraglottic swallow requires an effortful breath-hold, whereas the supraglottic swallow requires a breath-hold with no extra effort. The reason for the extra effort in the super supraglottic maneuver is to ensure glottal closure. Endoscopic inspection has revealed that adults (both normal swallowing and dysphagic) may not completely close the glottis during a breath-hold maneuver without vocalization or increased effort. Figure 10-4 demonstrates the difference in glottal closure patterns between a simple breath-hold maneuver and a forced or effortful breath-hold maneuver. Figure 10-4A demonstrates the glottal closure pattern associated with a simple breath-hold maneuver (i.e., supraglottic swallow). The primary feature is the horizontal (right–left) movement of the arytenoid cartilages and vocal folds to close the airway. When complete, this pattern may be effective in accomplishing airway protection during swallowing attempts. However, endoscopic inspection has shown that more than one third of adults who are asked to perform a simple breath-hold maneuver do not completely close the glottis. Adding force to the breath-hold maneuver increases the probability of complete glottal closure. Figure 10-4B demonstrates the glottal closure pattern associated with a forceful breath-hold maneuver (super supraglottic swallow). Note that in addition to the horizontal closure pattern observed in the supraglottic swallow, the arytenoids move anteriorly, approximating the **petiole** of the epiglottis. The result of this movement is more complete closure of the entire supraglottis, rather than closure at the level of the vocal folds only. Of interest is the observation that these two glottal closure patterns (horizontal and anterior) reflect stages in glottal closure in the normal swallow. As demonstrated in the accompanying videotape (Crary and Groher, *Video Introduction to Adult Swallowing Disorders,* Butterworth-Heinemann), slow-motion analysis of the normal swallow reveals that the glottis is initially closed by the horizontal (medial) movement of the vocal folds. Subsequently, before laryngeal elevation, the arytenoid cartilages move forward to approximately the petiole of the epiglottis. These closure patterns are reflected respectively in the supraglottic and super supraglottic swallow maneuvers.

Physiologic effects of the supraglottic swallow maneuver have been assessed in both normal and dysphagic adults. Different studies report varied findings ranging from no difference between the supraglottic swallow and a control (normal) swallow, to prolonged airway closure, increased anterior laryngeal movement, increased tongue-base movement, and increased PES opening. The super supraglottic swallow has been noted to increase the degree of laryngeal elevation during swallowing and to have a positive impact on swallowing

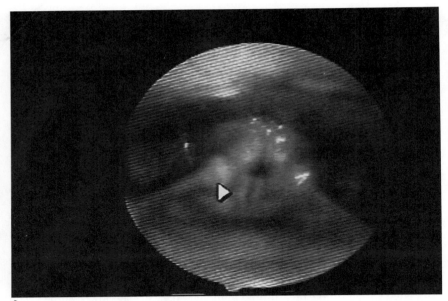

A

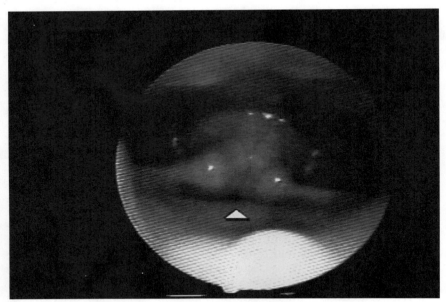

B

FIGURE 10-4 Laryngeal configurations associated with normal breath-hold (**A**) and effortful breath-hold (**B**). These photos were taken from video.

coordination. Unfortunately, most reports providing this information include only small numbers of subjects. In this regard, clinicians should consider using these findings as guidelines for evaluating change in swallowing in individual patients that may result from application of these maneuvers. These maneuvers are also considered compensatory, in that they may contribute to improved swallowing function when applied correctly. Evidence suggesting that they have a lasting positive impact on swallowing once the maneuver is no longer applied (rehabilitative function) is limited.

Prolonging the Swallow: The Mendelsohn Maneuver

The Mendelsohn maneuver is achieved by asking the patient to suspend the swallow at the peak of hyolaryngeal elevation and pharyngeal contraction and to prolong this posture for a couple of seconds before relaxing and allowing the swallowing tract to return to the preswallow position. The intent of this maneuver is to prolong and extend hyolaryngeal elevation. This has been a consistent finding in studies examining biomechanical and physiologic changes in the swallow created by this maneuver. Some investigators have suggested that this maneuver also prolongs PES opening; however, this is not a consistent finding across studies of normal swallowing. Figure 10-5 presents a lateral fluoroscopic view of a swallow in the resting position and during the elevated and contracted position of the Mendelsohn maneuver.

The Mendelsohn maneuver has been used extensively as a therapy technique and may serve both compensatory and rehabilitative functions. The compensatory function is indicated in studies that report reduced postswallow residue and aspiration when using this maneuver. The rehabilitative function is indicated in those studies that report improved swallowing function following use of this technique and without dependence on the technique. In general, positive outcomes in swallow function resulting from application of the Mendelsohn maneuver in dysphagia therapy have been reported.

One clinical concern about this technique is that it can be difficult to teach patients how to complete the maneuver. Some authors have advocated telling patients to squeeze their throat muscles at the top of the swallow and hold that squeeze for several seconds. Other authors have advocated using touch to instruct the patient—first having the patient touch the clinician who is modeling the technique and then having the patient touch his or her own throat to provide tactile feedback. Still others have advocated using adjunctive biofeedback, primarily **surface electromyography,** to provide patients with immediate physiologic information on muscle activity during attempts at the maneuver. Each of these may have pros or cons for an individual patient. Another clinical concern regarding this maneuver is that, if it is performed correctly, the prolongation of the swallow will increase the **apneic phase of the swallow.** This prolonged cessation of respiration may be contraindicated in patients suffering from respiratory disease or with severe incoordination between swallowing activity and respiration.

Effortful Swallow

The effortful swallow technique, sometimes referred to as the *hard swallow* or the *forceful swallow,* represents an attempt on the part of the patient to increase the force applied to the bolus from structures within the swallowing mechanism.

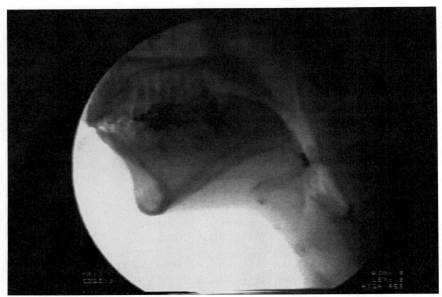

A

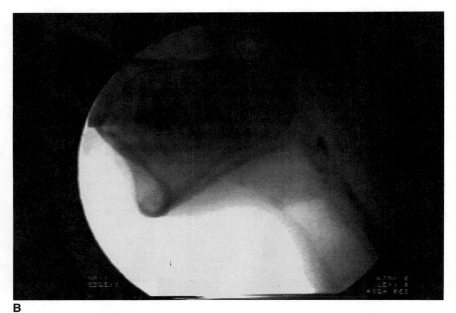

B

FIGURE 10-5 Pharyngolaryngeal configuration at rest **(A)** and with the Mendelsohn maneuver **(B)**.

Two presumptions have been offered in reference to this swallowing adjustment: (1) barring deficit within the PES, increasing effort results in improved bolus flow and less residue postswallow, and more specifically, (2) increasing effort during swallowing increases base of tongue movement. This second point relates to what some investigators have termed the *lingual driving force* created by the posterior and downward movement of the tongue base during the swallow. No reports have evaluated the functional impact of increased effort during swallowing; however, reports have addressed the physiologic impact of this "maneuver" on swallowing in both normal and dysphagic adults. In one report, adults increasing effort during swallowing demonstrated reduced hyoid-mandibular distance preswallow, reduced maximal hyoid excursion during swallow, and reduced laryngeal elevation during swallow. These observations may relate to the same common denominator—a higher position of the hyolaryngeal complex before the swallow onset. If the hyoid bone, and by attachment, the larynx, rests higher in the pharynx before a swallow, each of the observations listed previously would be realized. The distance between the mandible and the hyoid bone is reduced by a higher resting position, and thus the hyoid bone has a potentially smaller range of excursion during swallowing. Likewise, because the larynx is attached and follows the hyoid bone during swallowing, the degree of laryngeal elevation may be reduced if the initial preswallow position is higher. In a second, larger report, hyoid bone superior movement (and by attachment, laryngeal excursion) was greater in healthy adults who completed effortful swallows compared with regular swallows. No suggestion was made concerning the apparent disagreement with the prior, smaller study. Perhaps differences in procedure (combined manometry and fluoroscopy versus fluoroscopy combined with oral pressure assessment) or differences in bolus size (3 versus 10 ml) might account for these differences. Nonetheless, a common finding between these two studies was that swallowing biomechanics were altered when swallowing effort was increased. In addition to degree of movement, oral pressures (tongue to palate) and several measures of duration (hyoid anterior excursion, laryngeal vestibule closure, PES opening) were increased in the effortful swallow condition.

In patients with pharyngeal dysfunction, the effortful swallow had no impact on the number of misdirected swallows or on the degree of pharyngeal residue; however, it did reduce the depth of penetration of swallowed material into the larynx and trachea. In this respect, the effortful swallow was similar to the chin-tuck maneuver.

To encourage patients to use the effortful swallow technique, the clinician's instructions may vary from "swallow hard" to "when you swallow squeeze all your muscles." One limitation of this technique is that it may be difficult to ascertain whether the patient actually did swallow with increased effort or whether the increased effort came from the appropriate muscle groups. At least two options are available to clinical practitioners to address this scenario: (1) Use instrumental measures that evaluate pressure or muscle recruitment or (2) rely on a more indirect, but functional monitor such as change in a specific swallowing characteristic. Examples of the first option include pressure-measuring devices placed within the mouth to measure effort exerted by the tongue against the palate during swallowing or the use of surface electromyography to evaluate the degree of muscle activity during swallowing. Examples of the second option include a reduction of postswallow throat clearing, suggesting less (or less severe) material in the airway or decreased postswallow expectoration, suggesting less oral residue. Comparing a patient's performance with and without applying a maneuver can be a valuable clinical strategy.

Tongue-Holding or Masako Maneuver

Some question may exist regarding the clinical use of the so-called Masako maneuver. A little background may elucidate this situation. The posterior pharyngeal wall has a tendency to "bulge" forward during swallowing, contacting the tongue base and thus creating a pressure source to help push the bolus through the pharynx. When the tongue base is not able to move posteriorly toward the pharyngeal wall, and if the pharyngeal wall is physiologically capable, it may increase the degree of anterior "bulge" in a presumed attempt to compensate for the reduction in tongue base—pharyngeal wall contact. The initial clinical observations were made from a group of patients with oral cancer who demonstrated anchoring of the anterior tongue, limiting posterior movement of the tongue. These individuals demonstrated anterior bulging of the posterior pharyngeal wall. Subsequently, healthy young adults were asked to perform a maneuver that attempted to mimic the anterior anchoring of the tongue. These healthy subjects held the anterior tongue (slightly posterior to the tongue tip) between the teeth while swallowing. Fluoroscopic inspection indicated that with this maneuver during swallowing, the healthy adults demonstrated an increase in the extent of anterior bulging of the posterior pharyngeal wall.

Swallowing with this anterior tongue-hold maneuver appears to contribute to increased anterior movement of the posterior pharyngeal wall during swallowing; however, at least three negative consequences of this maneuver during swallowing have been identified: (1) reduced duration of airway closure, (2) increased postswallow residue, and (3) increased delay in the initiation of the pharyngeal component of the swallow. In some patients, each of these alone or in combination could contribute to an increased possibility of airway compromise (penetration or aspiration). This observation necessitates a cautionary note applied to this maneuver: the Masako or tongue-hold maneuver should not be used with a bolus. Furthermore, currently no evidence supporting the clinical application of this maneuver exists beyond the observations mentioned previously. It may have clinical application in cases in which an increase in anterior bulging of the posterior pharyngeal wall at the level of the tongue is desired. However, type of patient, specific dysphagia characteristics, and specific anticipated outcomes need to be further detailed in reference to this technique.

Isotonic/Isometric Exercise: The Shaker Exercise

What has become known as the Shaker (pronounced "shaw–keer") exercise is an activity intended to improve opening of the PES by increasing the strength of certain muscle groups that contribute to PES opening. The suprahyoid (and other) muscles cause the hyolaryngeal complex to move up and forward, exerting an upward and anterior pull on the PES. This is an important physiologic component to PES opening. Strengthening these muscle groups is expected to have a positive impact on PES opening with the use of these mechanisms. The exercise program used to strengthen these muscles requires the patient to lie supine and raise the head (but not the shoulders) sufficiently to see the toes.

This head posture is maintained for a prescribed period and repeated on a prescribed schedule. Results of this exercise are limited but do suggest increase in target muscle activity and improvement in PES opening and a subsequent reduction in postswallow residue and aspiration. Contraindications for this activity may include cervical spine deficits, reduced movement capability of the neck (as in some head/neck cancer patients), or possibly, cognitive limitations or other factors that might contribute to poor compliance with the prescribed routine. In addition, at this point, subject descriptions in clinical reports are limited. Practitioners must await larger and more detailed studies before this therapy becomes more widely applicable.

Thermal-Tactile Application

Thermal-tactile application is perhaps one of the grandparents of dysphagia therapy. It has been used for years and has been revised and revisited in many treatment-related and swallow physiology studies. One theory behind this technique (and other sensory-based techniques) is that provision of a sensory stimulus before a swallow attempt may serve as an alerting mechanism to the nervous system and may help prepare the swallowing mechanism for the subsequent swallow. Cold, tactile stimuli are presented to the anterior faucial pillars by stroking these sites with a cold laryngeal mirror (taken from a cup of ice). The primary outcome measure of success for this technique is a reduction in the delay in the initiation of swallowing, primarily the pharyngeal phase. By logical reasoning then, this technique may be suitable for patients who demonstrate a delay in the initiation of the pharyngeal aspect of swallowing. Studies evaluating functional benefits from this technique, such as reduction in aspiration, have not provided positive results. Thus this technique may be applicable for patients demonstrating delays in swallowing activity but not for patients who demonstrate airway compromise. Unfortunately, available literature does not provide more extensive patient selection criteria, and results across both normal and dysphagic adults are mixed in the presence and extent of timing changes following application of this technique.

One negative aspect of the application of this technique may be the dose required to facilitate change. Although limited, available research suggests that effects from thermal-tactile stimulation are most evident with extensive repetitions of stimulation to the anterior faucial pillars. The sheer burden of extensive repetition may make this technique pragmatically inappropriate for some patients or in certain environmental situations.

Adjunctive Behavioral Therapies: Biofeedback

Many of the maneuvers discussed in this chapter require motor learning on the part of the patient. Furthermore, many of these swallowing adjustments represent novel motor patterns and may be difficult to learn. Application of biofeedback as an adjunct to therapy may be valuable in enhancing the rate of motor learning, resulting in reduced time in therapy. Biofeedback has been shown to be facilitatory in teaching new movements, unfamiliar movements, or movements that are otherwise difficult to monitor. Many swallowing therapy maneuvers fit into one or more of these categories.

Various forms of biofeedback may be applicable to swallow therapy. Having the patient watch the swallow attempts on the monitor during a fluoroscopic examination has been advocated as a way to teach certain maneuvers. Obviously, this is a short-term application, but it is potentially valuable for certain patients. Endoscopic biofeedback has been suggested as a mechanism to teach appropriate breath-hold maneuvers such as the supraglottic and super supraglottic swallows. Clinical reports have shown that endoscopic biofeedback reduces therapy time and enhances outcome. If available, endoscopic biofeedback may be a valuable adjunct in teaching certain maneuvers. Less invasive than either fluoroscopy or endoscopy is the use of cervical auscultation as a biofeedback approach. Having patients listen for specific sound patterns may facilitate more rapid change in the swallowing pattern. Finally, multiple reports have advocated using surface electromyographic (sEMG) biofeedback as an adjunct in dysphagia therapy. This form of biofeedback has been used to teach relaxation, strengthening, and coordination activities. Studies specific to dysphagia therapy have suggested that this form of biofeedback can reduce the amount of time in therapy while producing favorable outcomes, even in patients with chronic dysphagia.

Whatever form of biofeedback is chosen, it is important for clinical practitioners to remember that biofeedback alone is not known to be therapeutic. As an adjunct to a well-conceived plan of therapy, judiciously applied biofeedback can have a positive impact. The key word seems to be *adjunct*. The key concept is "what change is intended to be facilitated by biofeedback."

FINAL COMMENTS ON USING EVIDENCE

Information is not the same as evidence. Evidence is information that has been filtered systematically through scientific processes and that meets minimal standards of rigor. Early in this chapter, clinically relevant questions regarding application of evidence were discussed. Although levels of evidence were not provided for each technique discussed in this chapter, most techniques are supported by some degree of evidence (primarily case reports, case-control studies, or small cohort studies). This is a start and, as a profession, we are moving toward obtaining stronger evidence for our therapeutic endeavors. Clinicians can focus on simple but important questions in helping choose appropriate clinical interventions. Perhaps the first consideration is whether information is published in credible journals or other formats. If so, does more than one publication exist? Replication of clinical findings is an important component of building supportive evidence. If information is not obtained in a published format, is it based on referenced publications? This initial step provides some indication of the degree of scientific review. The levels of evidence described previously in this chapter can be referenced when trying to decide how strong the evidence supporting a given technique might be. However, given the overt recognition that most techniques have not been subjected to the highest levels of evidence, clinical practitioners still need to rely on some system to evaluate whether a given technique might be appropriate for a specific patient. The following questions may help in this regard. These questions are not meant to be exhaustive, rather they are intended as a starting point from which clinicians may evaluate information and evidence on therapy techniques when trying to decide whether they are appropriate for specific patients. When reading available literature to assist in choosing a therapy technique, clinicians must ask themselves the following questions:

1. Were the patients in the study similar to my patient?
2. Was the technique described in sufficient detail so that I may use it in the same way?
3. Was the technique applied in an environment similar to the environment in which I practice (e.g., hospital, outpatient clinic, long-term care facility)?
4. Does the technique require technology that is available (or not available) to me?
5. Are the outcomes obtained in the study the same (or similar) to those I want to obtain for my patient?
6. Were failures and reasons for failure described in the study?
7. Do I have the clinical skills to apply this technique as it is described in the study, or is specific training required?
8. Is the technique pragmatically appropriate for my patient and environment (e.g., does it have time demands or intensity demands that exceed the reality of my workload or my patient's endurance or compliance)?

TAKE HOME NOTES

- Evidence-based practice offers practitioners a systematic approach to improve clinical practice and enhance the care of individual patients. This approach involves finding, evaluating, and using scientific information.
- Although most evidence supporting dysphagia intervention is not at the strongest levels, evidence does exist that can guide clinical practice and facilitate improved individual patient care.
- Compensatory techniques are intended to be used short term and provide an adjustment to the swallowing pattern that has immediate positive impact on safe swallowing. Rehabilitative techniques may not have an immediate impact, but contribute to reorganization of the impaired swallow, leading to improved functional swallowing once the technique is no longer applied.
- Many factors should be considered before applying a therapy technique. These factors may address the technique, the patient, the environment, and/or the clinician. Not all techniques have been studied to the point of providing information on all of these factors. Clinical practitioners should consider many factors, even in the face of limited evidence, before applying a given therapy technique.
- The functional impact of some therapy maneuvers is overtly evaluated during imaging studies. Others may require additional, adjunctive procedures (such as biofeedback) to evaluate, teach, and monitor the impact of the technique.

CASE EXAMPLE

The patient is a 70-year-old man who is 2 years post–brainstem stroke. He is receiving all nutrition by a percutaneous endoscopic gastrostomy tube, but is attempting to swallow some liquids with reported intermittent success. Fluoroscopic swallowing evaluation indicates reduced pharyngeal contraction, reduced hyolaryngeal movement, and reduced PES opening. No aspiration is noted, and the patient is able to clear residue effectively by throat clearing and expectoration.

In searching for information on how to best approach the chronic dysphagia in this patient, the clinician discovers three published articles describing therapeutic experiences with chronic dysphagia in brainstem stroke. Two of the articles are from different centers and use slightly different approaches, although both incorporate a modification of the Mendelsohn maneuver and both use sEMG biofeedback to teach this technique and monitor physiologic progress. The third article is a summary of a retrospective outcome study from one of the centers reporting on a larger number of patients. Not all of these patients suffered brainstem stroke.

Interpreting the Evidence The strength of evidence in this case is a level IV. These studies are case series using the patients as historical controls. Both include a small number of patients and are retrospective. The fact that different centers have reported similar results with similar patient groups reflects a degree of replication that strengthens the evidence.

An initial question is whether the patients reported in these studies resemble this clinician's patient. In large part, this depends on the detail of description of the patients in the articles and on the evaluation completed on the clinician's patient. This is essential if the clinician is to apply the described techniques to his patient. Do the evaluation results, functional eating profile, chronicity, and other descriptive characteristics of the published patient groups resemble this patient? Was the technique applied in an environment similar to that in which the clinician is seeing his patient? If this patient matches the published descriptions, the technique may be appropriate for him.

A second question might be whether the outcomes described in the articles were the same as those the clinician wants to achieve for his patient. How were these outcomes measured? Does the clinician understand and can he use similar outcome measures? Did these outcome measures make sense in terms of the problems being presented by his patient?

The next question the clinician asks might be, "Did I understand the treatment technique?" This depends on the degree of description within the publications. Did the therapy protocol make sense? Were specific steps described, including how often the techniques were applied and how many repetitions were used for each application? In this specific instance, sEMG biofeedback was used. Therefore is this equipment available to the clinician? Does he have the skills to use this technology or can he acquire them in a time frame that will allow him to use them with this specific patient? Was the application of the biofeedback to the therapy technique clearly explained in the articles? Can the patient use this technique as described in the articles?

A final consideration from the publications might be whether failures were reported and described. Clinicians are acutely aware that not all patients improve to the same degree. It is important to know which patients in therapy studies did not improve and, if possible, why they did not improve.

It may not be possible to address all these questions based on published literature. Practitioners are faced with the task of addressing as many of these questions as possible before application of any technique. The closer the individual patient fits the profile of published descriptions, the stronger the argument in favor of applying that specific technique.

CHAPTER TERMS

apneic phase of the swallow the time portion of the swallow in which respiration is ceased corresponding to glottal closure

compliance/noncompliance compliance and noncompliance refer to the extent to which a patient follows a treatment plan

efficacy addresses the question of whether a treatment can work; efficacy is established in the controlled circumstances of clinical research; it is different from effectiveness, which reflects more the impact of a treatment in ordinary clinical circumstances

intraluminal technically meaning "within the lumen or tube"; in the current context, this term refers to within the opening of the esophagus

petiole technically meaning "a slender stalk or stem"; in the current context, the term refers to the narrow base of the epiglottis within the laryngeal vestibule

surface electromyography a technique by which the electrical activity of moving muscles is detected by electrodes applied to the skin over the muscle groups of interest

SUGGESTED READINGS

Ali GN et al: Influence of cold stimulation on the normal pharyngeal swallow response, *Dysphagia* 11:2, 1996.

Bisch EM et al: Pharyngeal effects of bolus volume, viscosity, and temperature in patients with dysphagia resulting from neurologic impairment and in normal subjects, *J Speech Hear Res* 37:1041, 1994.

Bulow M, Olsson R, Ekberg O: Videomanometric analysis of supraglottic swallow, effortful swallow, and chin tuck in health volunteers, *Dysphagia* 14:67, 1999.

Bulow M, Olsson R, Ekberg O: Videomanometric analysis of supraglottic swallow, effortful swallow, and chin tuck in patients with pharyngeal dysfunction, *Dysphagia* 16:190, 2001.

Castell JA et al: Effect of head position on the dynamics of the upper esophageal sphincter and pharynx, *Dysphagia* 8:1, 1993.

Chang FY et al: Alteration of distal esophageal motor functions on different body positions, *Hepatogastroenterology* 43:510, 1996.

Crary MA: A direct intervention for chronic neurogenic dysphagia secondary to brainstem stroke, *Dysphagia* 10:1, 1995.

Crary MA, Groher ME: Basic concepts in surface electromyographic biofeedback in the treatment of dysphagia: a tutorial, *Am J Speech Lang Pathol* 9:116, 2000.

Drake W et al: Eating in side-lying facilitates rehabilitation in neurogenic dysphagia, *Brain Injury* 11:137, 1997.

Ekberg O: Posture of the head and pharyngeal swallowing, *Acta Radiol Diagn* 27:691, 1986.

Ertekin C et al: The effect of head and neck positions on oropharyngeal swallowing: a clinical and electrophysiologic study, *Arch Phys Med Rehabil* 82:1255, 2000.

Fujiu M, Logemann JA: Effect of a tongue holding maneuver on posterior pharyngeal wall movement during deglutition, *Am J Speech Lang Pathol* 5:23, 1996.

Fujiu M, Logemann JA, Pauloski BR: Increased postoperative posterior pharyngeal wall movement in patients with anterior oral cancer: preliminary findings and possible implications for treatment, *Am J Speech Lang Pathol* 4:24, 1995.

Hind JA et al: Comparison of effortful and noneffortful swallows in healthy middle-aged and older adults, *Arch Phys Med Rehabil* 82:1661, 2001.

Huckabee ML, Cannito MP: Outcomes of swallowing rehabilitation in chronic brainstem dysphagia: a retrospective evaluation, *Dysphagia* 14:93, 1999.

Johnsson F et al: Influence of gravity and body position on normal oropharyngeal swallowing, *Am J Physiol* 269:G653, 1995.

Kahrilas PJ et al: Volitional augmentation of upper esophageal sphincter opening during swallowing, *Am J Physiol* 260:G450, 1991.

Lazarus CL: Effects of radiation therapy and voluntary maneuvers on swallow functioning in head and neck cancer patients, *Clin Commun Disord* 3:11, 1993.

Lazzara G, Lazarus CL, Logemann JA: Impact of thermal stimulation on the triggering of the swallowing reflex, *Dysphagia* 1:73, 1986.

Lewin JS et al: Experience with the chin tuck maneuver in postesophagectomy aspirators, *Dysphagia* 16:216, 2001.

Logemann JA et al: The benefit of head rotation on pharyngoesophageal dysphagia, *Arch Phys Med Rehabil* 70:767, 1989.

Logemann JA et al: Super-supraglottic swallow in irradiated head and neck cancer patients, *Head Neck* 19:535, 1997.

Logemann JA et al: Effects of postural change on aspiration in head and neck surgical patients, *Otolaryngol Head Neck Surg* 110:222, 1994.

Mendelsohn MS, Martin RE: Airway protection during breath holding, *Ann Otol Rhinol Laryngol* 102:941, 1993.

Ohmae Y et al: Effects of two breath-holding maneuvers on oropharyngeal swallow, *Ann Otol Rhinol Laryngol* 105:123, 1996.

Rasley A et al: Prevention of barium aspiration during videofluoroscopic swallowing studies: value of change in posture, *AJR Am J Roentgenol* 160:1005, 1993.

Rosenbek JC et al: Effects of thermal application on dysphagia after stroke, *J Speech Hear Res* 34:1257, 1991.

Rosenbek JC et al: Comparing treatment intensities of tactile-thermal application, *Dysphagia* 13:1, 1998.

Rosenbek JC et al: Thermal application reduces the duration of stage transition in dysphagia after stroke, *Dysphagia* 11: 225, 1996.

Sackett DL et al: Clinical epidemiology: a basic science for clinical medicine, 2 ed, Boston, 1991, Little, Brown and Company.

Shaker R et al: Augmentation of deglutitive upper esophageal sphincter opening in the elderly by exercise, *Am J Physiol* 272:G1518, 1997.

Shanahan TK et al: Chin-down posture effect on aspiration in dysphagia patients, *Arch Phys Med Rehabil* 74:736, 1993.

Tsukamoto Y; CT study of closure of the hemipharynx with head rotation in a case of lateral medullary syndrome, *Dysphagia* 15:17, 2000.

Welch MV et al: Changes in pharyngeal dimensions effected by chin tuck, *Arch Phys Med Rehabil* 74:178, 1993.

C H A P T E R 11

Swallowing Disorders and Ethics

FOCUS QUESTIONS

1 What are the basic principles of medical ethics?
2 Why does a swallowing specialist need to be informed on issues of medical ethics?
3 What is an Advance Directive?
4 How might treatment of dysphagia be affected by an Advance Directive?
5 What are the various types of feeding tubes?
6 What are the risks and benefits of tube feeding?
7 What does the clinician tell the aspirating patient who wants to continue to eat?

MEDICAL ETHICS

In 1991, Congress passed the Patient Self-Determination Act. The act established guidelines to allow patients to participate fully in decisions regarding their health care, particularly decisions that are made in circumstances of severe or terminal illness. It strives to establish a patient-physician interaction that allows both parties to balance individual morals and values against the known risks and benefits of proposed medical care. For example, patients might want to decide under which circumstances they want to be resuscitated or whether they want to be nourished by a feeding tube to sustain life. Counseling patients, families, and caregivers on the risks and benefits of tube feeding may involve the expertise of the dysphagia specialist.

Medical ethics is a subspecialty of medical care that brings together patients, caregivers, and nonmedical and medical professionals in an effort to make the best decision on a health care issue. The decision rests on the understanding that it is finalized by balancing data from individual and societal morals and values, evidenced-based medical knowledge, and legal precedent. When balance is not achieved, wherein one party is not in agreement with the plan of care, ethical dilemmas result. For example, a patient may not agree to the short-term use of a nasogastric feeding tube because of religious objections, although the medical team is convinced that it may save or prolong the patient's life. These dilemmas need to be solved and may be referred to the medical center's ethics committee. Solutions generally are possible with a rational analysis of the following: (1) how the patient came to establish his or her health care preferences; (2) the medical risks and benefits of a proposed intervention; (3) the burdens that medical intervention might bear on the patient and family; (4) the effect on the patient's and family's quality of life; and (5) any legal constraints, such as the patient being incapable of making an informed decision.

Advance Directive

The Advance Directive is a statement made by a person with decision-making capacity, indicating what his or her preferences are for receiving or not receiving medical treatment. Most often, it is specific to end-of-life decisions or to circumstances when an individual's medical condition is futile. Typically, there are two parts to the Advance Directive: a living will and a durable power of attorney for health care. The *living will* is a written request to forego some type of medical treatment in a terminal or irreversible medical condition. The *durable power of attorney for health care* appoints a person (**surrogate**) to act in the patient's behalf regarding end-of-life or irreversible conditions should the patient be in a state that he or she is not competent to make an informed decision. It is understood that the surrogate will have prior knowledge of the patient's desires, and therefore is acting in the patient's best interest.

TUBE FEEDING

Because most ethical dilemmas that the swallowing specialist faces center around the use or denial of tube feeding, it is important to understand the risks and benefits of this intervention. There are psychologic and medical risks and benefits to tube feeding.

There are two major categories of nonoral nutritional provision: enteral and parenteral. Nonoral feedings are sometimes collectively referred to as *hyperalimentation*.

Enteral Nutrition

The major types of enteral tube feeding include (1) nasogastric, (2) gastrostomy, and (3) jejunostomy. Specially prepared high-caloric formulas are delivered through the tube into the feeding site. They are delivered either from a syringe, from a plastic bag that hangs above the level of the tube site, or from a mechanical pump.

Nasogastric Tube. Tubes that go through the nose and into the stomach can be used to deliver nutrients or to suction unwanted secretions. Tubes that provide nutrition are called *nasogastric feeding tubes*. They range in diameter from 8 to 18 Fr. Usually, the larger the diameter, the stiffer and more uncomfortable the tube is in the nose and throat. Larger nasogastric feeding tubes are necessary for passing medications and pureed foods. They do not clog as much on these materials as do smaller-bore tubes. Smaller-bore tubes take thin, liquid formulas; sometimes are prone to clogging; and generally are more comfortable in the aerodigestive tract. Smaller-bore tubes that are weighted on the tip for ease of passage are called *Dobhoff™ tubes*. The nasogastric feeding tube is inserted through the nostril into the pharynx, through the pharyngo-esophageal segment into the esophagus, and finally, through the lower esophageal segment into the stomach. In some cases, it is passed beyond the stomach, through the pyloric valve, and into the jejunum. Typically, it is used in acute medical situations that render the individual unable to swallow or unable to sustain nutrition orally. A nasogastric feeding tube is used when the medical care team thinks that the patient's medical status has a good chance to improve in a short period. Although the length of time for its use is not prescribed, if a patient requires enteral feeding for longer than 3 or 4 weeks, another enteral feeding method normally will be selected. More permanent options that are still reversible include the placement of gastrostomy and jejunostomy feeding tubes. These tubes can be placed surgically (usually requiring general anesthesia) or endoscopically (requiring light anesthesia). Endoscopic placements are called **percutaneous endoscopic gastrostomy (PEG)** or **percutaneous endoscopic jejunostomy (PEJ)**.

Gastrostomy and Jejunostomy Tubes. The gastrostomy tube is placed directly into the stomach with the assumption that the digestive processes of the stomach are intact. Formula is passed through a catheter that sits on the outside of the stomach. If the stomach is not functioning, the feeding tube may need to be placed into the jejunum of the small intestine. Because the stomach is bypassed, specialized, predigested formulas are required for jejunal tube feedings. Some clinicians argue that jejunal placement reduces the risk of reflux of tube feeding into the pharynx, because the pyloric valve offers an additional barrier to retropulsion; however, the experimental evidence does not clearly support this contention. The medical risks and benefits of enteral tube feeding are summarized in Table 11-1.

Parenteral Nutrition

Parenteral nutrition is indicated when the gastrointestinal tract cannot be used because of medical complications such as **gastroparesis**, obstruction, or bleeding. Total parenteral nutrition is a specialized formula that most commonly is delivered into a central vein (subclavian or internal jugular). Although there are potential medical complications from this therapy, patients can be supported nutritionally on this formula for 4 to 6 weeks if necessary. Peripheral parenteral nutrition is a form of nutritional support that is delivered through a peripheral vein. Because of potential medical complications, this therapy can be used effectively only for 7 to 10 days.

TUBE FEEDING USE

The three most common reasons for placing a feeding tube include the following: (1) The patient has been unable to sustain nutrition orally, although the swallow response is safe; (2) the patient requires sufficient calories on a short-term basis to overcome an acute medical problem; and (3) the patient is at risk for tracheal aspiration if he or she is allowed to eat orally.

The decision to place a feeding tube can be controversial and may precipitate ethical dilemmas that involve the entire medical care team. In general, there are no clear guidelines for long-term feeding tube placement, and in most cases, the wishes of the patient or family guide the decision. For patients who are too ill to swallow, and whose medical status is expected to improve, the decision to provide enteral feeding is apparent, and usually without controversy. The decision is more difficult for the patient who is eating safely, but cannot eat enough, particularly if the patient has an advance directive that states an unwillingness to be tube fed. In this situation, the patient may be putting himself or herself at

Table 11-1	*Medical Risks and Benefits Associated with Enteral Tube Feeding*

RISK	BENEFIT
NASOGASTRIC	
Uncomfortable	Easy insertion
Poor cosmesis	No anesthesia
Distends PES and UES; may	Can be small bore; well tolerated
promote reflux	Good short-term nutrition
Nasal ulceration	Patient can eat with tube in
Sinusitis	
Delays swallow	
May trigger vagal bradycardia	
GASTROSTOMY	
Requires surgical placement	Good long-term option
Infection and care at tube site	Out of visual sight
Tube may fall out	Easy tube replacement
Reflux if stomach fills too fast	Easily removed
Diarrhea	Patient can eat with tube in
JEJUNOSTOMY	
Requires surgical placement	May reduce reflux
Needs continuous drip feeding	Out of visual sight
Requires hospital visit if dislodged	Good nutrition if stomach
Intolerance of special formula	not available
PERCUTANEOUS ENDOSCOPIC GASTROSTOMY OR JEJUNOSTOMY	
Aspiration during procedure	Inserted under local anesthesia
Infection at tube site	Generally well tolerated
Potential for reflux	OR time not needed

OR, Operating room; *PES,* pharyngoesophageal segment; *UES,* upper esophageal segment.

medical risk from the consequences of undernutrition and dehydration. Placing a feeding tube in a patient who is at risk for tracheal aspiration to avoid the consequences of that aspiration (e.g., life-threatening aspiration pneumonia) also is controversial. The literature suggests that for patients with chronic, terminal diseases, a gastrostomy or jejunostomy does not reduce the incidence of aspiration pneumonia. Furthermore, the literature suggests that they do not prolong life beyond expected limits. For patients with longer life expectancies, or for patients with dementia who are not interested in eating, tube feeding may extend their life without undue risk. The decision to place a feeding tube in a patient needs to be carefully considered, and the patient's or surrogate's wishes must be weighed against the medical risks and benefits.

ASPIRATION PNEUMONIA

Aspiration pneumonia is a lung infection that may result from three primary sources: aspiration during swallowing, including saliva; retention of swallowed contents that eventually are aspirated; or aspiration of gastroesophageal contents. Physical signs include shortness of breath with a rapid heart rate, acute mental confusion, incontinence, and infection. Some patients develop fever and an increase in sputum with cough. It has been shown that elderly patients may have aspiration pneumonia with few of these overt signs. A chest radiograph may show diffuse **infiltrates**, usually in the posterior and right segments of the lung. If the source of the infection is thought to be related to oropharyngeal dysphagia, the patient is kept from eating while antibiotics are used to treat the infection. If the source is thought to come from the gastrointestinal tract, medications and posturing may be used to reduce the threat of recurrence.

Risk Factors for Aspiration Pneumonia

Not all patients who aspirate material into the lung develop aspiration pneumonia. For example, some patients frequently aspirate their saliva and do not become ill. This may be explained by the fact that their oral hygiene is sufficient to not allow bacteria to colonize and, in turn, infect the lung tissue. When material is misdirected into the upper airway during swallow attempts, the first line of defense is cough at the level of the vocal folds. If the cough is sufficiently strong, most of the material may be expelled back into the pharynx to be swallowed, while only a small amount enters the trachea below the level of the vocal folds. Even if material does get into the lung, it may trigger a secondary cough response that further protects the lower airway spaces. Specialized cells in the tissue of the lung work to engulf, absorb, and transport foreign fluid and food out of the lung spaces. Other cells produce a chemical reaction that neutralizes aspirants that are acidic. For example, the acid in gastric reflux is particularly virulent in the lung field. The upper and lower airway defense systems are most active when the patient's immune system is strong. Therefore patients with an acute medical problem or older patients with chronic, multiple medical problems may be at increased risk for the development of aspiration pneumonia.

Although the data are not strong, some preliminary evidence suggests that certain clinical signs are predictive of aspiration, whereas other variables (mostly historical) are more predictive of who will develop aspiration pneumonia. In other words, not all patients who aspirate will develop aspiration pneumonia. Interestingly, there are no data to support the concept that those clinical indicators from the clinical examination that predict aspiration also predict aspiration pneumonia. Clinical signs from the physical examination that are associated with aspiration were discussed in Chapter 7. These signs include dysarthria; dysphonia; a wet, gurgling vocal quality; and coughing on secretions. Clinical signs that suggest (although the evidence is not unanimous) risk for developing aspiration pneumonia are seen in the following patients: (1) those who are advanced in age and have a compromised immune system; (2) those with oral bacteria colonization (poor oral hygiene) who aspirate; (3) those who are bedfast; (4) those who cannot self-feed; (5) those who have multiple medical diagnoses and are taking many medications, especially those that sedate; (6) those with a prior history of aspiration pneumonia; and (7) those with respiratory impairment such as chronic obstructive pulmonary disease. Although not yet tested formally, it may be assumed that patients who evidence many of these features are at greater risk for the development of aspiration pneumonia.

NONMEDICAL RISKS AND BENEFITS

In addition to being informed about the medical risks associated with tube feeding, clinicians, patients, and caregivers also need to be informed of the nonmedical risks and benefits to make an informed decision regarding whether enteral feedings are in the patient's best interest.

Nonmedical Benefits

Some dysphagic patients continually struggle to maintain sufficient nutrition and hydration orally. Similarly, caregivers who are assisting patients in their nutritional needs also may be burdened by the fact that maintaining nutritional levels is a challenge. Family members often are troubled by the fact that their loved one is losing weight. Weight loss leads to a decrease in energy levels, and mobility may be decreased. Poor nutritional levels also may precipitate mental confusion. All of these factors are viewed by the patient and family as a diminution in the quality of life. This realization often is accompanied by situational depression. Providing the patient with sufficient calories by enteral feeding may relieve the burden of trying to maintain nutrition orally. In turn, the quality of life for the patient and caregiver improves. Lost functions may return, because nutrition and hydration levels have a chance to return to normal. Although the patient and caregiver may have to familiarize themselves with the mechanics and care of the enteral feeding route, there are some instances in which enteral feeding can provide both physical and psychologic relief from dysphagia.

Nonmedical Risks

Patients who no longer eat by mouth, or who must consider not eating by mouth, may feel threatened because they are losing one of life's basic pleasures. Thus social withdrawal and depression may be a consequence of their decision. Patients who are demented and require enteral feeding may have to be sedated and physically restrained, because they attempt to dislodge the feeding tube. Being sedated and restrained while taking enteral feedings often is seen as a risk, because it further erodes the patient's quality of life.

ETHICAL DILEMMAS

A myriad of ethical dilemmas may develop when doctors and patients consider tube feeding. Ethical dilemmas usually are the result of the patient or caregiver not agreeing with, or failing to understand, the medical care team's plan. In most cases, dilemmas can be resolved by reviewing the circumstances that led to the decision. Such a review entails an in-depth discussion among the key members of the medical team, the patient, and the family that is especially devoted to conflict resolution. If the dilemma is not solved in this meeting, a request for resolution is sent to the medical center's ethics committee. In general, this committee is composed of physicians, nurses, a psychologist or social worker, a chaplain, and a member from the community. The swallowing specialist or dietitian may be asked to be a part of the committee if the issues require his or her expertise. In some cases, a clinician who deals extensively with swallowing disorders is a member of the committee.

Ethical issues in medicine surface for a number of reasons. First, the patient or family member is not convinced that the medical advice he or she has received has sufficient evidence to support the conclusions. Second, determinations of the best course of care, as well as who the final arbiter of making that decision is, may not be clear. For example, the patient may have been told by his or her attending physician what the best course of care would be, but also received an opposing opinion from an outside consultant whom the patient trusts. Third, the medical care team and the patient may have personal biases that interfere with rational decision making. Fourth, it may not be clear who is acting in the patient's behalf and whether that person is acting in accordance with the patient's best interest. Finally, it may not be clear what the patient or surrogate views as a desirable outcome to the dilemma.

It is the task of the medical ethics committee to resolve ethical dilemmas that surface when the medical team recommends a feeding tube and the patient or family refuses or when the patient wants a feeding tube and the medical care team thinks it is not necessary. The committee performs a thorough, nonbiased review of the medical and nonmedical risks associated with tube feeding in an effort to resolve the dilemma. In most cases, the committee does its best to honor the patient's wishes within accepted legal and ethical boundaries.

AN ETHICAL DILEMMA

One of the most commonly encountered dilemmas that the swallowing specialist faces is the patient who is a known aspirator and has decided that under no circumstances does he or she want a feeding tube. A dilemma may arise when the medical team has decided that the risk of developing aspiration pneumonia during continued oral feeding is greater than the risk of developing aspiration pneumonia with enteral feeding. If the medical care team is convinced that the patient and family understand all of the risks of continued oral feeding, they most likely will honor the patient's wishes under the Patient Self-Determination Act and let the patient continue to eat. At this point, a number of dilemmas may surface. The physician who allowed the patient to continue to eat, although he or she was convinced that it was not in the patient's best interest, may feel that he or she is sacrificing his or her professional responsibility. Furthermore, the physician may feel liable for legal action if the patient develops aspiration pneumonia and expires. In this case, it is important that specific documentation is in the medical record regarding the medical team's recommendations and the patient's refusal of those recommendations. Some institutions require the patient to acknowledge that he or she has refused the medical team's advice in a separate written document. These documents have not been challenged in the courts, so their validity remains questionable.

The swallowing specialist whose evaluation might have helped the team make the decision that oral feeding was contraindicated also may believe that his or her professional ethics are at risk, particularly if he or she is asked to continue to assist the patient by providing the "safest" way to feed. Some clinicians might argue that they would be assisting the patient toward his or her own demise and that they would be libel to court action should the family choose to do pursue it. In this case, the clinician has the right to sign off the case and pass it to another colleague who may have a different perspective. Another colleague may believe that he or she can provide safe feeding instructions without compromise to his or her personal ethics. In most cases, the swallowing specialist will provide additional care if he or she is convinced that the patient and family were fully informed of the continued risk, and if it was properly documented in the medical record.

TAKE HOME NOTES

- Medical ethics is a subspeciality of medical care that brings together patients, caregivers, and nonmedical and medical professionals in an effort to make the best decision on a health care issue. It is driven by a congressional mandate called *the Patient Self-Determination Act.*
- An Advance Directive is a statement made by a patient that provides guidance to health care professionals regarding the patient's wishes for treatment or no treatment in certain medical circumstances.
- The two broad categories of nonoral feeding are enteral and parenteral.
- The major enteral feeding routes are nasogastric, gastrostomy, and jejunostomy.
- Feeding tubes do not necessarily reduce the risk of aspiration pneumonia, nor prolong life.
- Not all patients who aspirate will develop aspiration pneumonia. Some clinical factors are more predictive than others at identifying which patients who aspirate will develop pneumonia.
- Ethical dilemmas regarding the use and acceptance of tube feeding can result between the patient and the medical care team. Most of these dilemmas can be resolved with a review of the patient's wishes and a review of the medical evidence.
- Professional ethics can be threatened if a patient refuses to follow medical advice. Asking another professional to assume the care of the patient is within a practitioner's right.

CASE EXAMPLE

A 55-year-old man had been in a nursing home for 10 years with an unknown, progressive disease of the basal ganglia. It affected all of the muscles of the head, neck, and limbs. Because he was counseled early in the disease that it would progress and lead to a premature death, he executed an Advance Directive that stated he did not want any heroic measures when he became terminally ill. This included a statement that he did not want to be fed through a tube in his stomach. His disease progressed to the point where he could not produce intelligible speech because of weakness in the muscles of articulation. To compensate, he used an electronic communication board. He continued to eat orally, but choked violently at every meal as the nurses were feeding him. At the time of the consult with speech pathology, he had been treated for six episodes of aspiration pneumonia in the previous 18 months. His videofluorographic swallowing examination showed aspiration on all bolus volumes and types, ranging from thin liquid to a semisolid. He was capable of transferring the bolus from the mouth to the pharynx. He was asked numerous times if he wanted to change his mind regarding the possibility of feeding tube placement to perhaps lessen the risk of developing pneumonia, but he refused.

The entire issue came to a head when the nursing assistants banded together and said they did not want to continue to feed him because they felt they were contributing to his death. The patient did not have a family member in the vicinity who might have been available to provide feeding assistance. A consult was sent to the ethics committee to resolve the dilemma.

The ethics committee reviewed the entire medical history and established that the patient fully understood his medical condition. The committee found him competent to make decisions about his health based on what the medical care team had communicated regarding the risks and benefits of continued oral feeding and the risks and benefits of tube feeding. It was clear from the speech pathologist's report that dietary compensations and behavioral swallowing treatment strategies were not successful in reducing the patient's risk of aspiration. It also was apparent that the nurses were not willing to be cooperative with his feeding, leaving the patient at nutritional risk. After extensive discussion, the surgeon on the committee asked if it would be prudent to perform an elective laryngectomy, effectively separating the airway and food tract to avoid the risk of aspiration. This would sacrifice vocal fold function. Because the patient's speech was already unintelligible, it seemed like a reasonable option to sacrifice voice for swallow safety. This option was explained to the patient, who agreed to the procedure.

CHAPTER TERMS

gastroparesis paralysis of the stomach muscles affecting the digestive process
infiltrates deposition of materials into a cell, tissue, or organ
percutaneous endoscopic gastrostomy (PEG) the insertion of a feeding tube
    into the stomach with endoscopic guidance
percutaneous endoscopic jejunostomy (PEJ) the insertion of a feeding tube
    into the jejunum with endoscopic guidance
surrogate a substitute, especially an emotional substitute for another

SUGGESTED READINGS

Blustein J: The family in medical decision making. In Monagle JF, Thompson DC,
    editors: *Health care ethics,* Gaithersburg, Md, 1998, Aspen.
Emanuel LL, Emanuel EJ: The medical directive: a new comprehensive advance care
    document, *JAMA* 261:3288, 1989.
Fein AM: Pneumonia in the elderly: special diagnostic and therapeutic considerations,
    Med Clin N Amer 78:1015, 1994.
Feinberg MJ et al: Aspiration in the elderly, *Dysphagia* 5:61, 1990.
Finucane TE, Christmas C: Aspiration pneumonia, *N Engl J Med* 344:1869, 2001.
Finucane TE, Christmas C, Travis K: Tube feeding in patients with advanced dementia:
    a review of the evidence, *JAMA* 13:1365, 1999.
Griggs B: Nursing management of swallowing disorders. In Groher ME, editor: *Dysphagia:
    diagnosis and management,* Boston, 1997, Butterworth-Heinemann.

Groher ME: Ethical dilemmas in providing nutrition, *Dysphagia* 5:102, 1990.

Groher ME: The detection of aspiration and videofluorography, *Dysphagia* 9:147, 1994.

Langmore SE et al: Predictors of aspiration pneumonia: how important is dysphagia? *Dysphagia* 13:69, 1998.

Lazarus BA, Murphy JB, Culpepper L: Aspiration associated with long-term gastric versus jejunal feeding: a critical analysis of the literature, *Arch Phys Med Rehabil* 70:46, 1990.

Lo B, Dornbrand L: Understanding the benefits and burdens of tube feedings, *Arch Intern Med* 149:1925, 1989.

Rabeneck L, McCullough LB, Wrary NP: Ethically justified, clinically comprehensive guidelines for percutaneous endoscopic gastrostomy tube placement, *Lancet* 349:496, 1997.

Rudberg MA et al: Effectiveness of feeding tubes in nursing home residents with swallowing disorders, *J Paren Enter Nutr* 24:97, 2000.

Sharp HM, Genesen LB: Ethical decision-making in dysphagia management, *Am J Speech Lang Pathol* 5:15, 1996.

Silver KH, VanNostrand D: The use of scintigraphy in the management of patients with pulmonary aspiration, *Dysphagia* 9:107, 1994.

Index

Page references followed by "f" indicate figures, "t" indicate tables, and "b" indicate boxes.